Psychiatric Emergencies

How to Accurately Assess and Manage the Patient in Crisis

DEBORAH ANTAI-OTONG

ISBN: 1-55957-991-9

PESI HealthCare strives to obtain knowledgeable authors and faculty for its publications and seminars. The clinical recommendations contained herein are the result of extensive author research and review. Obviously, any recommendations for patient care must be held up against individual circumstances at hand. To the best of our knowledge any recommendations included by the author or faculty reflect currently accepted practice. However, these recommendations cannot be considered universal and complete. The authors and publisher repudiate any responsibility for unfavorable effects that result from information, recommendations, undetected omissions or errors. Professionals using this publication should research other original sources of authority as well.

Continuing Education Self Study Credit Available: PESI HealthCare provides self study credit for this publication. Please see the information contained in the back of this book for details.

**For information on other PESI HealthCare products
and seminars, please call 800-843-7763.**

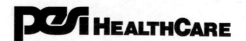

www.pesihealthcare.com

Acknowledgments

I would like to thank my best friend and lifelong supporter, my husband Okon who tends to bring out my creativity and support my eagerness to learn and write. I also want to thank my mother Gladys, for her unique wisdom, patience, and love. Finally, I want to extend my appreciation to Mike Conner and Patti Johnson of PESI HealthCare, who provided a supportive and encouraging atmosphere that enabled me to travel extensively and do programs on psychiatric emergencies. These experiences along with eager audiences gave me the courage to write this book.

About the Author

Deborah Antai-Otong, MS, RN, CNS, NP, CS, FAAN is a clinical, educational, organizational and legal consultant. She is also a certified mediator and an professional communicator. She is a nationally sought speaker on various topics including psychosocial, addiction, depression, anxiety disorders, dementia, psychopharmacology and psychiatric emergencies. Ms. Antai-Otong is also a motivational speaker and expert on diverse topics including conflict resolution, mediation, team building, anger management, dealing with difficult people, workplace violence and assertiveness training. She has numerous referred nursing and medical publications, including *Journal of Psychiatric Research, Psychopharmacology, Neuropharmacology, Federal Practitioner, Nursing, American Journal of Nursing, Journal of Addictions Nursing, Advance for Nurse Practitioners,* and *Geriatric Nursing.* She is a manuscript reviewer and member of numerous editorial boards including *Journal of Addictions Nursing, Advance for Nurse Practitioners* and *Clinical Nurse Specialist.* She is the author/editor of several books including *Psychiatric Nursing: Biological and Behavioral Concepts* (Delmar Thomson Learning), *Psychiatric Emergencies* (PESI) and co-author of *Decision-Making in Psychiatric and Psychosocial Nursing* (BC Decker). She is a psychotherapist and has extensive experience working with clients experiencing depression, grief, anger management, early childhood trauma and borderline personality disorder. Her clinical expertise includes psychiatric emergencies, medication management, crisis intervention, workplace violence, and psychiatric consultation and employee assistance. She received her MS in psychiatric mental health nursing and BS from Texas Woman's University and post-master certificate as a Psychiatric Mental Health Nurse Practitioner from the University of Texas at Arlington.

Contents

Contents

Tables

Introduction

1

The treatment of psychiatric inpatients has undergone dramatic changes in the managed care era. Managed care, changes in health care delivery systems, and decreasing access to mental health services are increasing the prevalence of psychiatric emergencies. Moreover, managed care has narrowed the parameters of hospitalization resulting in an increased utilization of care in emergency departments and the community-based settings (Allen, Currier, Hughes, Docherty, et al, 2001; Christodulu, Lichenstein, Weist, Shafer & Simone, 2002; Povar, Blumen, Daniel, Daub, Evans, et al, 2004; Wickler, Lessler, Travis, 1996). Frequently, only the suicidal, homicidal or seriously ill clients with complex and major psychiatric disorders are being hospitalized. Cost-containment pressures, shorter lengths of stay, and a lack of opportunities to form therapeutic alliances contribute to poor treatment compliance and increase the risk of relapse and psychiatric emergencies. Psychiatric emergency refers to a severe disturbance of mood, thought or behavior that needs immediate attention. This generally means that the client presents to an Emergency Department (ED) or other health care settings with complaints of acute symptoms, psychological and/or physical distress that overwhelms his or her present coping capacity.

The emergency department or psychiatric triage unit often serves as an entry to the health care system due to problems with access, lack of knowledge regarding mental health help, or concerns about the stigma attached to seeking help at mental health centers. These factors often result in clients seeking care during a time of crisis resulting in increase use the ED. High use of emergency departments and shorter lengths of stay place tremendous pressures on providers in diverse clinical settings. Most health care facilities offer 24-hour staffing with mental health professionals who can evaluate, diagnose, provide crisis intervention, stabilize, and triage or make appropriate referrals. Other facilities are inadequately staffed with mental health professionals and provide an initial assessment and disposition. Facilities inadequately staffed with mental health professionals often misdiagnose and make inappropriate referrals (Garbrick, Levitt, Barrett, & Graham, 1996).

The complexity of client needs and tremendous changes in mental health delivery systems make it imperative for health care providers to sharpen their clinical skills. Expert clinical skills in the management of psychiatric emergencies offer the client quality mental health services and immediate access to assessment and treatment. Emergency mental health care plays an important role in the continuum of psychiatric health care. Because of the impact of managed care on mental health delivery systems, the prevalence of psychiatric emergencies and provision of care have become an integral aspect of psychiatric services (Allen, et al, 2001; Nicholson, Young, Simon, Fisher, & Batemen, 1998). Major advantages of emergency mental health services include expediting access to treatment of the mentally ill client; thwarting a crisis or decreasing its potential deleterious effects; and reducing incarceration of the mentally ill client by making appropriate dispositions.

Triage or psychiatric emergency decisions determine client placement at appropriate levels of care often parallel the client's presentation and include the following

- danger of harm to self or others
- level of functioning, and capacity for self-care
- severity of psychiatric symptoms
- ability to comply with treatment recommendations

- comorbid psychiatric and physical disorders
- quality and availability of support systems
- client and family preferences
- available resources

Overall, the mental health continuum of care comprises vast individual elements or services and extends from acute inpatient to diverse community-based settings. Regardless of treatment setting, the appropriate identification and management of psychiatric emergencies requires an array of clinical expertise that offers the client appropriate, expeditious and quality mental health services.

Selected Readings

Allen, MH; Currier, Hughes, DH; Reyes-Harde, M; Docherty, JP; Expert Consensus Panel for Behavioral Emergencies. (2001). *Postgraduate Medicine (Special Edition)*, 1–88.

Christodulu, K; Lichenstein, R; Weist, MD; Shafer, ME & Simone, M (2002). Psychiatric emergencies in children. *Pediatric Emergency Care, 18*, 268–270.

Fawcett, J (2000). Are psychiatric emergencies on the increase? *Psychiatric Annals, 30*, 232.

Garbrick, L; Levitt, MA; Barrett, M; & Graham, L (1996). Agreement between emergency physicians and psychiatrists regarding admission decisions. *Academy of Emergency Medicine, 3*, 1027–1030.

Nicholson, J; Young, SD; Simon, LJ; Fisher, WH; & Batemen, A (1998). Privatized Medicaid managed care in Massachusetts: Disposition in child and adolescent mental health emergencies. *Journal of Behavioral Health Services Research, 25*, 279–292.

Povar, GJ; Blumen, H; Daniel, J; Daub, S; Evans, L; Holm, RP; Levkovich, N; McCarter, AO; et al, (2004). Ethics in practice:

Managed care and changing health care environment. *Annals of Internal Medicine, 141,* 131–136.

Simon, SI (1998). Psychiatrists' duties in discharging sicker and potentially violent inpatients in the managed care era. *Psychiatric Services, 49,* 62–67.

Scott, RL (2000). Evaluation of a mobile crisis program: Effectiveness, efficiency, and consumer satisfaction. *Psychiatric Services, 51,* 1153–1156.

Wickler, TM; Lessler, D; & Travis, KM (1996). Controlling inpatient psychiatric utilization through managed care. *American Journal of Psychiatry, 153,* 339–345.

Principles of Psychiatric Emergencies

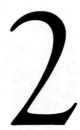

Safety Considerations

Managing psychiatric emergencies begins with appreciating the importance of personal and staff safety. Personal safety often eludes health care providers because of their need to take care of others often at the expense of compromising their own safety. During the initial assessment of the client presenting in crisis, health care providers must gather as much information as possible through client records, discussions with referring agencies, family members and of course the client. This often involves discerning if the client has a history of violence, including domestic violence, past arrests, and past and present legal problems. This process also involves asking referring agents about the client's history of violence towards self and others.

Prior to taking a client into a closed area also requires exploring one's work area for items that may be used as weapons, such as scissors. Clinicians must position themselves between the client and an exit. Waiting until the client becomes aggressive before insuring this position is an often ignored safety issue even for the experienced mental health professional. Health care providers must also be able to muster assistance in the event that help is needed. Recognizing that all clients have the potential to become violent is basic to creating a safe work environment.

A summary of key safety issues is:

- Make personal and staff safety a priority!
- Realize that violence can occur anywhere
- Position yourself between the client and exit
- Gather as much information as possible about the client, including history of violence and legal problems

Developing a Sense of Severity of the Clients' Symptoms

Another area of concern for clinicians dealing with psychiatric emergencies is differentiating an emergent situation from an urgent or non-emergent situations. The assessment of the client's presenting symptoms requires identifying a imminent danger situation from a non-dangerous situation. (*See* **Table I:** Psychiatric Triage and Process for a further discussion of these categories.)

The foremost challenge for health care providers dealing with psychiatric emergencies is determining what is an emergent versus non-emergent psychiatric situation. Once an emergent situation is determined, decreasing noise, activity and anxiety in the client and staff reduce the client's symptoms. Table I offers some strategies for discerning the nature of the client's presenting symptoms and possible interventions. Along with determining the nature of the client's presenting symptoms and possible interventions and dispositions, the mental health provider must also create a therapeutic relationship that afford the client safety, reassurance, empathy, and a supportive environment.

Table I: Psychiatric Triage Determination and Process

Category	Rationale	Initial Intervention(s)

Emergent	Requires immediate attention:
	
	• unstable or abnormal vital signs
	• impending alcohol withdrawal
	• violent or threatening behaviors
	• drug toxicity
	• acute drug-related side effects, such as acute dystonia,
	• suicide attempts (high lethality level)
		• Assess physical status and rule out medical conditions and make appropriate medical or psychiatric referral
		• Initiate psychosocial and/or pharmacological interventions
		• Assess mental status
		• Initiate appropriate physical controls including:
		  • verbal de-escalation
		  • restraints
		  • 1:1 observation
		  • seclusion

Urgent	Requires attention, but does not constitute an emergency: • bizarre behavior • acute agitation • suicidal/homicidal risk • intoxication • evaluations for commitments • suicide gestures	(same as above)

Non-emergent	Situation does not require immediate attention, but client must be assessed in a timely manner. Examples include:
	  • situational disturbances
	  • mild to moderate anxiety
	desire "to talk"
	medication questions
		• Afford a courtesy and reassurance
		• Inform client of estimated time he/she will be seen
		• Offer alternatives, such as keeping present mental health appointments
		• Address other treatment issues when appropriate

Areas of interest that create the appropriate environment include providing ample space, privacy, minimal noise or stimuli. **Ample space** refers to one that reduces the client's anxiety and distress that is about leg's length. It important to realize the clients experiencing crisis and psychological distress are very sensitive to environmental stimuli. Leg's length is a comfortable distance that reduces anxiety and severity of symptoms. It also provides a safe distance for the health care provider. An exception to this rule is the client who presents in a manic episode of bipolar disorder who may be intrusive and get into the clinician's comfort zone. It is important for the clinician to ensure safety by maintaining a safe distance.

Privacy is essential to forming therapeutic interactions, however, it should never compromise one's personal safety. Talking to the client in an open area, particularly if the client is under the influence of intoxicants or cognitively impaired, is crucial to maintaining staff safety. Certainly, when the client is mentally stable, privacy is crucial to the data gathering process and enables the clinician to obtain personal information. Ample space and privacy along with creating an environment with **minimal noise or stimuli** also reduce the client's anxiety. A seclusion room can also be used, but the client's vital signs must be assessed prior to placing him or her in this type of enclosure. Restraints may be necessary long enough for an in-depth evaluation, particularly when the client is unknown or etiology of symptoms is indecisive. This is particularly important when clients are experiencing delusions, delirium or acutely agitated. Making sure that the room is **well lit** also reduces illusions and other environmental misperceptions that may increase the risk of violent or aggressive behaviors. Creating a safe and non-threatening environment also involves determining how much time is required to manage a particular psychiatric emergency.

Clinicians often find themselves dealing with a large number of clients experiencing psychiatric emergencies. Effort to manage the clients' care in a **timely manner** challenges them to make quick and important decisions about the client's presenting symptoms and appropriate disposition. Most psychiatric emergencies require about 30 to 45 minutes to assess and manage. An exception to this time frame is working with children, individuals requiring crisis intervention and those who are cognitively impaired. Gathering pertinent information from various resources can also facilitate timeliness. Moreover, psychiatric emergencies must be managed expeditiously to minimize further deterioration, restore health, initiate appropriate treatment, and return the client back to a previous or higher level of functioning. Specific time for seeing clients presenting in a psychiatric emergency must be individualized. Individualized and client-centered approaches must determine time required assessing the client's presenting symptoms, level of dangerousness to self and others, and appropriate disposition. Ordinarily, child and adolescent emergency situations and geriatric emergencies, particularly with severe cognitive deficits require more time than others. An exception to this premise is the suicidal or depressed client who requires crisis intervention.

Crisis intervention is an important part of psychiatric emergency care. It provides the client with immediate emotional support and a problem solving process and helps the client explore options for dealing with the present crisis.

Summary of Strategies for Creating an Appropriate Environment include:

- Provide ample space, at least leg's length
- Afford privacy, but not at the risk of compromising personal safety
- Minimize noise and environmental stimuli
- Make sure the room is well lit
- Deal with the situation in a timely manner

Legal and Ethical Considerations

3

Prior to providing psychiatric interventions, the clinician must understand basic psychiatric emergency management principles that include the previous discussion. A final principle is understanding mental health care and legal-ethical considerations. Major areas include the right to care, confidentiality, informed consent, emergency petition, the right to refuse treatment and documentation.

A. *Right to Treatment*—Clinicians must safeguard the client's right to obtain and participate in their treatment. Clients presenting with psychiatric emergencies are entitled to care and treatment. Clinicians must assess the clients to discern an emergent situation from a non-emergent situation. Treatment must be provided according to the standards of care established in the community and duty to protect the client and others from potentially dangerous behavior.

B. *Confidentiality* is an obligation of clinicians that is necessary to foster a therapeutic clinician-client relationship. Information is shared verbally or recorded. Laws governing confidentiality vary, thus clinicians must be cognizant of laws governing their state practice.

C. *Informed consent* is a dynamic process that informs and educates the client and significant other about the purpose, benefits and potential adverse effects of treatment. Informed consent stems from the fundamental belief that clients should be able to have control over their bodies. More importantly, the informed consent is a legal requirement and affords clinicians with an opportunity to establish a therapeutic relationship with the client and or significant others. Only people who are competent may give informed consent.

D. *Competency* refers to the ability to perform a specific act. Under law all adults are considered legally competent to consent to treatment unless they are legally declared incompetent or temporarily incapacitated. Certainly, the client who presents with delirium, grossly psychotic, demented or under the influence of intoxicants is probably incompetent to make decisions. (In these situations, efforts to obtain consent for treatment must obtain a competent informed consent for treatment from family members.) In situations where the client is dangerous, consent issues are less relevant because most state laws permit treatment against his or her will. *Legal incompetency* refers to the status of persons who have been declared incompetent in a court of law or *to minors*.

E. *Emergency petitions* are being used by law officers who escort clients experiencing acute psychiatric symptoms to the ED. Frequently, police officers have the authority to emergency petition these clients who require emergent psychiatric intervention, such as suicidal or violent behaviors. The process of obtaining this petition varies across the country, but most have criteria for initiating emergency petitions. Clinicians must be cognizant of federal and statutory laws that govern their practice and guidelines to initiate emergent treatment of clients with mental disorders.

F. *Right to Refuse Treatment*—Clinicians must ensure that no barrier interferes with a client's right to make treatment decisions. Yet when the client refuses a treatment due to delusions or suicidal intent and the refusal poses a substantial threat to his or her or other's well being and integrity, emergency interventions may be justified.

For example, is a client (who has been of his neuroleptic for 2–3 weeks) who has brought to the ED by police officers after his mother calls 911. Additionally, his mother reports that he is hearing voices that are telling him to stab her and himself, yet he refuses medications in the ED. This scenario is an exception because obviously he poses a threat to himself and others, unless sedated. By treating this client over his objections is acting on behalf of the community and the client and his mother.

The *decision to initiate treatment,* such as medications, against the client's will requires supportive documentation to substantiate the act according to legal standards of the state.

G. *Documentation* provides a record of the client's presentation and process and rationale that guided the clinician's decision making process, treatment, referral and disposition. Every record is a legal document and information entered into the client's record must be legible, accurate, and timely. This record also reflects a standard of care that is determined by what a competent mental health professional would do under similar circumstance. Additionally, the client's record includes the source of data—client, family, others—and serves as the basis of treatment. It should also include information about informed consent and health teaching. It is imperative to understand that information documented in the client's record can also serve as evidence in a court proceeding. Pertinent information required in the record includes:

a. Reasons for seeking treatment

b. Appropriate diagnosis and rationale for treatment that reflects sound clinical judgement

c. All consultations

d. Data source—client, family member, health care professionals, police officer, etc.

e. Results of examinations—mental status exam, pertinent physical and laboratory findings

f. Justification for making referrals/dispositions

g. All referrals—dates, times, contact person

h. All follow up instructions to family members and client: removal of weapons from home, written instructions regarding worsening symptoms or adverse drug reactions

i. Health education, informed consent for treatment

j. Information about client who refuses treatment—whether he/she understands the consequences or refusal

k. Record all interventions thoroughly—including desired and adverse responses

l. "No harm" or "safety agreements" and a list of community referrals, hotlines, ED, if suicidal ideations recur

H. *Duty to Warn.* Clinicians have a duty to protect the public from dangerous acts carried by their clients. The *duty to warn* is based on a case law from 1976, *Tarasoff v. Regents of the University of California.* This law established the clinician has duty to warn a person who is the target of a homicidal client. The basis of this law involves breaching confidentiality and protecting others by warning the possible victim. The application of this duty varies among states. Clinicians must be familiar with their own state laws.

I. *Duty to Protect.* One of the guiding principles of psychiatric emergency care is to protect the client's health and integrity. In cases where the client's decisions for treatment or refusal of treatment are deemed dangerous to self or others, the clinician may need to exert an emergency petition to prevent harm at the expense of the client's right to make a clinical decision.

J. *Children, adolescents and families in crisis.* Clinicians have the daunting task of evaluating mental health and substance abuse needs and preferences during emergency situations. Legal issues involving children and adolescents vary from state to state and may emerge during the initial evaluation or treatment and after the evaluation concerning mandatory reporting of suspected child abuse and duty to warn or protect or warn third parties from harm. Confidentiality and release of information is a major concern prior to, during and after the interview. Clinicians must familiarize themselves with statuatory laws that govern confidentiality, mandatory reporting and civil commitment.

Suggested Reading

Dubowitz, J; Giardino, A; & Gustavson, E (2000). Child neglect: Guidance for pediatricians. *Pediatric Review, 21,* 111–116.

Fortunati, FGJ & Zonan, HV (2003). Legal considerations in the child in the psychiatric emergency department. *Child and Adolescent Psychiatric Clinics of North America, 12,* 745–761.

Hendricks, AL & Barloon, LF (2003). Legal and ethical issues. In D. Antai-Otong (Ed.) (pp. 167-191) *Psychiatric nursing: Biological and behavioral concepts.* Clifton Park, NY: Delmar Thomson Learning.

Simon, RI (1999). *Concise guide to psychiatric and the law for clinicians, 2nd ed.* Washington, DC: American Psychiatric Press.

Simon, RI & Goetz, S (1999). Forensic issues in the psychiatric emergency department. *Psychiatric Clinics of North America, 22,* 851–864.

The Clinical Assessment: The Initial Interview

4

Initial Approach

Once personal and staff safety and an appropriate environment are ensured, the clinician must initiate the formal data gathering process that begins with the client interview. This process requires an ability to quickly assess the client's symptoms, make a provisional diagnosis, rule out medical conditions that mimic psychiatric disorders, and stabilize the client's condition. This process is often contingent on available time, severity and nature of the client's symptoms. Another factor that plays a role in this initial process is the availability of information from the client, family members or friends, police officers, and other health care providers.

Families play key roles in this process and may offer vital information, when appropriate, about the client's medical and psychiatric history, compliance, family dynamics and support systems. Clinicians must determine how to deal with family members, particularly when there are more than several. Encourage the client to identify specific family members or family members if the client is unable to make this decision. The clinician must also determine when it is appropriate to see the client with family or separately. Seeing the client and family together is the most expedient approach to this process, unless there is evidence of domestic violence or the client objects.

Focus of the Bio-Psychosocial Assessment

I. Reasons for seeking treatment at this time.

This information enables the clinician to determine the nature of the emergency and reasons for seeking treatment at this time. The chief complaint can also be used to develop a provisional differential diagnosis. Sometimes clients present with complaints of feeling depressed "for years" and have no idea of their reasons for presenting today. This data also provides important information about the client's insight about present symptoms and treatment outcomes. Questions such as:

> **"What's brought you in today?"** (information about the chief complaint and reasons for seeking treatment now).
>
> **"What are your expectations today?"** (information about the client's wishes, preferences and needs from his or her perspective that guide the clinician's decision making process).

The following are examples of situations that impact the assessment process:

  a. *Children and adolescents* are usually brought in by their parents who express concerns about their behavior or safety. An accurate diagnosis of psychiatric disorders in children and adolescents is often challenging. Adolescents are challenged by developmental crises related to hormonal and physical changes and psychosocial stressors that threaten their self-esteem and social adjustment to adolescence. Exploring possible diagnoses, nature of the child-parent relationship, level of family stress, comorbid conditions, family history of medical and psychiatric illnesses and developmental issues is helpful in making differential diagnoses in this age group. A family history of psychiatric disorders, including mood disorders in biologic parents, comorbid with panic disorders, predicts an increased incidence and more severe symptoms in the youth.

b. Cognitively impaired clients, such as those with various dementias may be brought in by concerned family members

c. Others may be brought in by law officers in handcuffs either acutely psychotic, intoxicated, or aggressive, seeking an evaluation

d. *Older adults* may be referred for psychiatric evaluations because of physical complaints that have no basis. Because of socialization issues, such as difficulty asking for help, these individuals may have difficulty expressing their fear of being labeled "crazy." Older adults may also be referred because of acute or chronic confusional or cognitive deficits. Because mental status changes in older adults are often caused by an array of factors, especially polypharmacy and other medical conditions, differential diagnosis is crucial and may be life-saving. Psychiatric emergencies in this age group require a calm, objective approach, and decisive action to manage the problem and prevent aggravation or worsening of symptoms. Efforts to rule out underlying medical disorders, such as delirium, dementia and alcohol withdrawal are critical to making a differential diagnosis.

Other pertinent information includes:

1. Identifying data; demographics

2. Determine if visit is voluntary or involuntary

3. History of presenting symptoms—onset, duration, what alleviates or precipitates symptoms

4. Past and present psychiatric history, including information about diagnoses, medications, side effects, compliance, prescribing health care provider, and the last appointment.

5. Alcohol or other drug use history including treatment and last use, history of blackouts, withdrawal syndromes and seizures, the impact it has had on their overall functioning, including legal problems

6. Current health status—current medications, including over-the-counter herbal medications, last physical examination, major medical problems, recent past head trauma or accidents

7. Family history—a brief statement about any medical and psychiatric history and treatment

8. Quality of current support systems and availability–include cultural considerations

   a. Social and work history—present relationships, employment

   b. Legal history—including probation, history of arrests, abuse, domestic violence

9. History of abuse or trauma—both as survivor and perpetrator

II. Mental Status Examination (MSE)

(During a psychiatric emergency this exam should be brief and documented)

   a. **General description**—appropriateness should be closely observed throughout the assessment and accurately documented as part of the general MSE. *Observe for signs of abuse—*

bruises or other signs of injury, neglect, and determine if client looks his or her stated age.

1. Behavior—appropriateness, level of activity, psychomotor and motor function
2. Appearance—appropriateness, grooming, dress
3. Attitude towards clinician—cooperative, uncooperative
4. Psychomotor behaviors—including involuntary movements, tremors, and tics

b. **Mood**—congruency with affect and thought content

c. **Affect**—appropriateness and congruency with thought content

- Apathy*
- Elation
- Depressed*
- Blunted*
- Sad

*may indicate frontal lobe disease or adverse drug reactions

d. **Speech/Language characteristics**—rate, tone, ability to articulate, pressured, spontaneity, fluency, volume, prosody (affective inflection)

- Dysarthria—difficulty in articulation*
- Dysprosody—loss of normal speech melody*
- Aphasia—disturbances in language input*
- Agraphia—a loss of an ability to write in cursive style*
- Alexia—a loss of previous reading ability*

*suggests underlying neurological disorder

e. **Perceptions**—the content of hallucinations or illusions and what precipitates or aggravates them

- Visual*
- Tactile*
- Olfactory*

*usually associated with underlying medical conditions, including drug intoxication and withdrawal

f. **Concentration and Attention**—carefully document the client's ability to attend to the interview

g. **Thought content**—delusions, phobias, suicidal/homicidal ideations, ideas of reference

h. **Thought processes**—refers to organization-loose association, racing thoughts, circumstantiality and tangentiality

i. **Sensorium and cognition**

1. Level of consciousness—alert, comatose, drowsy, sedated
2. Concentration and attention—may be affected by intense anxiety, hallucinations, depression and cognitive disturbances including delirium and dementia
3. Ability to abstract—higher brain function—proverbs are useful
4. Orientation

- Names
- Ages
- Present place
- Address
- City
- Day of week
- Date

5. Memory function

- Immediate recall—ask to name 3 unrelated objects and repeating them in 5 minutes
- Recent memory—ask to recall events over the past few days
- Remote memory—ask historical questions relevant to educational level and culture

j. **Judgment**—ask "what if questions"

k. **Insight**—degree of understanding about their illness and treatment

l. **Reliability**—refers to truthfulness and dependability

m. **Impulsivity**—refers to the ability to control aggressive impulses, often impaired in cognitive disturbances, personality disorders, and substance use

Clear and *concise* documentation of the mental status examination (MSE) is crucial to the evaluation of all clients presenting with psychiatric symptoms. This data must be legibly documented and is important for clinical and legal purposes.

III. Suicide and Homicidal Assessment

(*See* Chapter 5 for an in-depth discussion of the suicidal client)

a. Factors that increase the risk of suicide include:

- psychiatric disorders—including mood disorders, panic disorder, schizophrenia
- substance use—intoxication and withdrawal
- significant losses
- history of attempts

- family history of attempts, mood disorders, alcoholism
- comorbid psychiatric and/or medical conditions
- age—older white males, adolescents
- race—white
- lack of quality support systems

IV. Differential Medical Diagnoses

All clients presenting with an onset of acute psychiatric symptoms require a basic medical evaluation. Clients with known histories of psychiatric disorders are at a greater risk of having a comorbid medical illnesses, cognitive disorders, and substance-related conditions. Clinicians often overlook medical disorders and presume that the client's symptoms are related to underlying psychiatric disorders. Making a differential diagnosis is of particular importance when clients present with symptoms or exacerbation of symptoms. Focused clinical psychosocial assessments provide information from the initial interview. Clinicians must integrate data gathered from the client, family and friends, facility records, and other health care providers and make accurate differential diagnoses. The presence of acute psychosis, agitation, or delirium does not justify deferring mental or physical status evaluations. A basic template of the evaluation process for clients presenting with psychiatric emergencies follows:

a. Current vital signs—abnormal suggest underlying medical, neurologic, or medication-related conditions

b. Physical observations—review of systems, medications and substance misuse

c. Last physical examination

d. Basic laboratory screens

- complete blood count with differential
- urinalysis

- alcohol (ethanol) blood levels
- hemoglobin and hematocrit
- chemistry profile—electrolytes, serum glucose (blood sugar)
- liver function tests
- renal function test—including urinalysis
- cardiovascular status—electrocardiogram
- drug toxicology screen—usually urine screen
- serum blood levels
- pregnancy test—childbearing women
- tests for sexually transmitted diseases when appropriate
- thyroid panel
- vitamin B_{12}, folate, and thiamine levels—especially in clients with a history of chronic alcoholism and older clients

Ultimately, data gathered from the psychosocial assessment and physical screening serves as the basis of the medical or psychiatric differential diagnosis. A medical diagnosis requires an immediate referral for a complete physical evaluation and treatment. Physical disorders, such as delirium or acute drug toxicity or adverse reactions require immediate attention to reduce further deterioration and stabilization.

V. Interventions

Interventions include psychosocial and pharmacological approaches. Interventions are based on the client's presenting physical and mental status; preferences; level of dangerousness, and age. Legal issues also guide the decision to implement specific interventions

VI. Disposition

The decision that underlies the referral and disposition process is in accordance with the client's physical and mental status, preferences, age and the client's ability to make sound treatment decisions. The quality of support system and access also play a role in where to refer the client for treatment, follow-up and transfer. For instance, the client who presents with a substance-related disorder and is stable will most likely be referred to a drug treatment program. A woman who is battered and acknowledges that she is willing to leave her spouse, will be referred to a woman's shelter or "safe house."

In contrast, a man who is medically unstable will be treated for medical problems and hospitalized for further evaluation and stabilization (i.e., severe alcohol withdrawal syndrome)

VII. Malingering

A final discussion of the psychosocial assessment process is incomplete without mentioning the importance of ruling out malingering. *Malingering* refers to voluntary production and presentation of false or marked distorted physical or psychiatric symptoms. Normally, the external motivation for malingering involves three major reasons:

- avoidance of difficult or dangerous situations, responsibilities, or legal concerns.
- compensation, a place to stay for free room and board or "three hots and a cot."
- retaliation for a recent loss (Sadlock & Sadock, 2003)

The DSM-IV-TR (APA, 2004) suggest that clinicians should suspect malingering when the client's reasons for seeking treatment involve:

- legal issues—probation, referral from attorney for non psychiatric reasons

- profound discrepancy between the client's complaints and actual presentation (i.e., vague, over dramatized, subtle and subjective in nature)
- uncooperativeness during the evaluation period
- evidence of Antisocial Personality Disorder

Evaluation/Interventions/Disposition of the Malingering Client—The evaluation of these clients must be the same as others who present complaining of a psychiatric emergent situation. During the evaluation process the clinician must establish rapport, maintain a professional demeanor and avoid making judgmental remarks about their suspicions. Collaboration with other health professionals helps validate and confirm the client's presentation as malingering. Once the determination of malingering is made the clinician must make an objective referral and disposition.

Selected Readings

American Psychiatric Association (2000). *Diagnostic and statistical manual of mental disorders, 4th edition, text revision.* Washington, DC: American Psychiatric Association.

Antai-Otong, D. (2003). *Psychiatric Nursing: Biological and behavioral concepts.* Clifton, Park, NY: Delmar Thomson Learning.

Axelson, DA & Birmaker, B (2001). Relation between anxiety and depressive disorders in childhood and adolescence. *Depression and Anxiety, 14,* 67–78.

Berenson, CK (1998). Frequently missed diagnoses in adolescent psychiatry. *Psychiatric Clinics of North America, 21,* 917–926.

Felker, B; Yazel, JJ; Short, D (1996). Mortality and medical comorbidity among psychiatric patients: A review. *Psychiatric Services, 47,* 1356–1363.

Kennedy, GJ; Onuogu, E & Lowinger, R (1999). Psychiatric emergencies: Rapid response and life-saving therapies. *Geriatrics, 54,* 38–46.

Korn, CS; Currier, GW & Henderson, SO (2000). Medical clearances of psychiatric patients without medical complaints in the emergency department. *Journal of Emergency Medicine, 18,* 173–176.

Olshaker, JS; Brown, B; Jerrard, DA; et al. (1997). Medical clearance and screening of psychiatric patients in the emergency department. *Academy of Emergency Medicine, 4,* 124–128.

Othemer, E; Othmer, JP & Othmer, SC (1998). Brain functions and psychiatric disorders. *Psychiatric Clinics of North America, 21,* 517–566.

Sadock, BJ & Sadock, VA (2003). *Synopsis of Psychiatry, 8th edition.* Baltimore, MD: Williams & Wilkins.

Suicidal Behaviors 5

Risk Factors: Adults

Acute Risk Factors and Diagnoses

Roughly one-third of clients experiencing a psychiatric emergency complain of suicidal or homicidal ideation or both. Predicting suicide remains a challenge to mental health professionals because of the potential legal consequences and liability concerns that make this an important issue. It is impossible to accurately predict suicide. The prevalence of suicide in the United States has remained constant for some time, at about 12 per 100,000 (McCraig & Strussman, 1997; Peters, Kochanek, & Murphy, 1998). Approximately 5% of persons in the community have attempted suicide at least once (Kessler, Borges & Walters, 1999). The most consistent demographic findings associated with risk for suicide include, being male, older than 45, white, living alone, and having a chronic medical condition. Completed suicides are most likely to occur in men over age 60, who use lethal means, such as firearms. A preponderance of research data suggest that more than 90 percent of adult suicides suffer from a major mental or emotional disorder (Antai-Otong, 2003; Harris & Barraclough, 1997; Fawcett, Clark, & Busch, 1993).

Predictability

The primary goal of assessing and treating the suicidal client is to keep the client alive; however, predicting it is perplexing. Hospitalization is an option, but the constraints of managed care principles challenges clinicians to explore other options, such as crisis intervention and day treatment. Moreover, hospitalization is often an unacceptable option to the client and family.

Among potential predictors, that have emerged from retrospective studies, both large community-based autopsy studies and studies of psychiatric clients, the following are identified as risk factors:

- The subjects talked about suicide (directly or indirectly) within 6 months prior to his or her death
- Previous suicide attempts
- Consultation with a physician within one month of the suicide (a non mental health specialist)
- Specific psychiatric disorders (*See* **Table II**)

Overall, these data suggest that even under ideal circumstances, the prediction of suicide is challenging.

Assessing for suicide

All suicide attempts and suicidal ideations must be taken seriously. Suicide is most likely to occur in clients experiencing major psychiatric disorders, such as major depression, chronic alcoholism, schizophrenia, and severe borderline personality disorder. Those clients presenting with comorbid psychiatric disorders are at a greater risk of suicide. The most critical to address in suicidal clients is the identification of acute suicidal risk. Because of shorter lengths of stay and pressures to facilitate the client's rapid improvement and hasty return to a previous level of functioning, clinicians must focus attention on the assessment and management of acute risk factors.

Table II: Psychiatric Disorders with High Suidice Risk Factors—Adults

- **Major Depressive Episode**—recurrent illness, postpartum mood disorders, and with delusions. Increase risk during the early course of treatment and with people with a history of being recently hospitalized for suicidality. (High risk with *abrupt improvement* with or without treatment.)
- **Bipolar disorders, Type I & II,** untreated
- **Alcoholism or substance misuse**—especially with comorbid disorders (i.e., major depression) and recent interpersonal losses
- **Schizophrenia**—young, male, early years of illness and previous history of attempt. More likely to occur during periods of improvement after relapse or during periods of depressed mood and hopelessness
- **Anxiety disorders**—panic disorder-especially with comorbid major depressive episode
- **Personality disorders**—particularly borderline personality disorder—especially with comorbid major depressive episode

General Assessment Considerations

Clinicians must make judicious clinical assessments and determine a safe and appropriate disposition of their clients and be cognizant of potential civil rights when considering committing clients presenting with high risk suicidal behaviors.

Cultural Factors

Clinicians must also recognize the impact of cultural factors on the acceptance of suicide as a coping strategy and continuously assess these issues. Moreover, despite the lower rates of suicides among various cultures, educational and socioeconomic factors tend to influence its prevalence. For instance, in a national study of data, (Stack 1998a, b) determined that for every year of education among black males, the risk of suicide increases 8%. In comparison, each year of education among white males is associated with a decrease of 2% in the risk of suicide.

Assessing the Suicidal Client

Major Considerations

1. Suicide is very personal, thus the clinician must approach the client in an empathetic and non-judgmental manner to establish rapport. It is imperative to ask direct questions about depression and suicide, especially in adults, and proceed from a general to specific perspective. For example, "What sort of things have been going on in your life that lead you to believe that suicide is the only option?"

2. Use a nonjudgmental and supportive approach

3. Establish rapport with the client

4. Use a suicide risk assessment that includes the following:

   • Suicidal ideations—"Are you having thoughts about killing yourself or others?"

   • Suicidal plan—Does the person have one?; provisions for being rescued; relevant mental status; details of plan

   • Level of lethality—is it lethal? Can the person die?

   • Suicidal intent and means—Does the client have the means of carrying out the plan?

   • Previous attempts—how many? What were the circumstances? When was the last time?

   • Is the client depressed or recently suffered a significant loss?

   • Does the client have a chronic or debilitating/terminal illness?

   • Does the client abuse or misuse alcohol or other substances?

   • What is the quality of the client's support system?

Note: If the client admits having suicidal ideations, with a plan and the means, another important question to ask is "What has stopped you from acting on these thoughts?" The client may have decided that this was not a good idea because of the effects suicide would have on family members and decide to seek help. In comparison, another client may have a gun in his mouth and is stopped by a significant other who rushes him to the ED. Regardless, of the client's response, an accurate and thorough evaluation must be performed to determine the lethality level, present stressors and treatment options.

- Personal and demographic risk factors for suicide. (*See* **Table III.**)

5. Asking about or discussing does not put ideas into the client's head. In fact, many clients welcome the opportunity to discuss this personal matter. Every client seen in a psychiatric emergency situation must be asked about suicide and homicide

6. All clients seeking psychiatric evaluations must be assessed for suicidal and homicidal risk. Clients often find it relieving to discuss their suicidal and/or homicidal ideations.

7. Clinicians must assess the client's level of hopelessness and be aware of its impact on the client refusing treatment, creating situations that negate help.

8. Clinicians must recognize their personal reactions to suicidal clients and their potential to result in premature termination of relationship and enhancing the client's sense of hopelessness.

9. Avoid using religion or other approaches to talk the client out of suicide. Overly zealous clinicians sometimes convey undue reassurances and a lack of empathy for the client's ideations. Allowing the client to express his or her thoughts and plans requires active listening skills and patience.

Table III: Risk Factors Associated with Suicide

High Risk Factors Associated with Suicide

1. **Previous suicide attempts or threats**—inquire about previous attempts, circumstances and treatment
2. **Presence of a suicidal plan and means**
3. **Age**—older males (65 years and older—*highest rate*)—especially those recently widowed or have been diagnosed with a debilitating medical problem
4. **Gender**—females attempt 3-4 times more than males.
   Males—2-3 times likely to kill themselves and females
5. **Race**—white males
6. **Psychosocial factors**
   - divorce
   - single
   - separated
   - widowed
   - those who live alone or are socially isolated
   - unemployed
   - lack of quality support systems
7. **Family history of suicide and/or attempts and positive psychiatric disorders, especially affective (mood) disorders**
8. **Health factors**
   - chronic pain
   - terminal illness
   - chronic disease
9. **Access to lethal means**—inquire (client and family) about weapons and removal from home
10. **Availability and quality of resources and support systems**
11. **A negative or pessimistic outlook on life, hopelessness**
12. **Recent psychiatric hospital discharge**

10. Evaluate the *suicide attempt* by asking the following questions:

- What were the circumstances of the act?
- What methods were used?
- What were the anticipated outcomes?
- Was the act impulsive or planned?

- Was the client sober or under the influence or withdrawing from alcohol or other drugs?

11. Assess client's present level of pessimissm or sense of hope-lessness, anger, agitation aggressive and impulsive traits.

Other Considerations

1. When triaging, indicate those clients who are in immediate danger and require prompt clinical attention.
2. Stabilize current or potential medical conditions
3. Provide adequate client safety

- confine and restrain
- remove dangerous objects
- monitor client appropriately
- use appropriate restraints—chemical (medications) and mechanical (as the last resort)

4. Take special *safety precautions* when dealing with clients who are intoxicated or in withdrawal—they are potentially violent because of cognitive deficits and disinhibition and profound agitation. Obtaining an alcohol blood level or other drug screens is helpful when justifying involuntary treatment or hospitalization.
5. Take *all* suicide threats seriously, even if they are deemed manipulative or chronic in nature.
6. Recognize that clients who exhibit a *sudden change* in their level of energy following a bout with depression must be thoroughly assessed for suicide

7. Consider hospitalization or an emergency petition if the client is an imminent danger to him or herself (if the client is *high risk* for suicide and *refuses hospitalization*, the physician becomes responsible for involuntary commitment in accordance with civil laws).

Legal and Ethical Considerations

Concerns about liability and ethical issues are an integral aspect of working with suicidal clients. Presently no professional standards exist for assessment of the risk for suicide or homicide (Beck & Baxter, 1998; Jacobs, 1999; Simon, 1999). Although present research does not delineate a specific standard of care for suicidal or homicidal clients, a thorough bio-psychosocial assessment and mobilization of resources enable clinicians to make appropriate dispositions and referrals.

The *major legal defense* for mental health professionals dealing with the suicidal clients is adequate documentation of the client's examination, a detailed history, diagnosis, suicide risk assessment, and the rationale for treatment options. Clinicians should rely on data from a thorough assessment rather than the client's denial of suicide intent and a willingness to "contract for safety." Presently, there is little basis for relying on the client's no harm contract during an acute psychiatric emergency or crisis. Involving and documenting family members and friends in this process must be an integral part of the decision-making process and treatment.

When the client is deemed suicidal and no bed is available or the client's family refuses to participate in an emergency petition, other steps must be initiated to reduce the risk of suicide. When immediate hospitalization is impossible, another alternative may be the client's home. In this case the physician must stress to family and friends that the potential for suicide remains high and provide them with written instructions to allay their anxiety and possible denial of the emergent situation. Special instructions to family and friends may include:

- Remove all dangerous objects from the home—guns, poisons, potentially harmful medications or household chemical, car keys
- Avoid leaving the client alone
- Observe the client continuously
- Administer prescribed psychotropic medications to manage the client's psychiatric symptoms
- Educate about desired and adverse drug responses
- Return to the ED or call 911 in the event of an emergency
- Keep telephone numbers of the local ED, crisis hotlines or other designated support systems

ED staff may also find themselves dealing with a suicidal client prior to hospitalization. When a client poses a danger to him or herself or others, measures to protect the client and staff must be initiated. Major measures for dealing with the suicidal client include:

- Remove potentially dangerous objects from the immediate area
- Provide one-to-one observation (constant observation)—even in the bathroom
- Administer adequate dosing of medications, such as anxiolytics/and or neuroleptics to relieve anxiety and agitation and observe for desired and adverse drug response

Simon and Goetz (1999) suggest the following guidelines for dealing with legal or forensic issues during psychiatric emergencies:

- Conduct a comprehensive bio-psychosocial evaluation to evaluate and manage the client's symptoms
- Obtain informed consent for treatment or procedures from the client or other health care decision makers
- Gather as much information about the client as possible and use as the basis of decision-making, plan of care and treatment

- Conduct a thorough suicide and violence risk assessment and make them the basis of clinical interventions
- Comply with basic safety measures and facility guidelines for dealing with potentially violent and aggressive clients
- Be cognizant of information about legal regulation (statutory and federal) of mental health practice, particularly those involving the evaluation and treatment of clients in the emergency department
- Secure legal consultation when the need arises regarding laws affecting client care (*See* Chapter 2 for an in-depth discussion of legal and ethical issues)

Treatment and Disposition

1. The disposition is contingent upon the client's present level and future potential for suicidality and ability to control suicidal impulses. The client presenting in an acute psychotic or intoxicated state will have difficulty controlling his or her impulses and poses a high risk of suicide.

2. The nature of external controls and available support systems accessible to the client. For instance, the older client who has been living alone, has family members who are willing to stay with him and administer medications is more likely to provide strong external controls. In contrast, a homeless client who has stopped taking medications and threatening to kill himself has poor external controls and requires inpatient hospitalization that affords external control against suicidal impulses.

3. The clinician's perception of the client suicide risk and its likelihood in the future. Risk factors must be considered.

4. Consider **crisis intervention** which offers immediate emotional support, enhances the client's problem solving skills, empowers

the client and reduces a sense of powerlessness and helplessness. Crisis intervention may involve seeing the client daily until the crisis is resolved or individualized to provide support during a stressful period. This intervention is ideal when:

- the precipitant is *clearly identifiable* (traumatic or sudden illness or death or separation)
- the client has *quality support systems* or self confidence to be able to return for crisis sessions
- the client has a history of a *moderate level of functioning* and is able to form a therapeutic relationship

Individuals who are *poor candidates* for crisis intervention include those with intense suicidal ideations, poor premorbid or lower level of functioning, or exhibit further deterioration rather than improvement after several sessions.

Practical Dispositions/Referrals

1. Outpatient referral including day hospital program, crisis mobile team, crisis center and home with family members
2. Crisis intervention—4–6 sessions for clients who are good candidates
3. Voluntary hospitalization if the client is medically or psychiatrically unstable after a high-lethality risk suicide attempt and has few resources or support systems. Decisions to hospitalize also depend upon the availability and quality of other treatment options and social support systems and resources.
4. Involuntary hospitalization

Documentation of Clinical Findings

Information about the suicidal client must involve careful documentation, both written and oral communication, about the rationale for decision-making surrounding discharge and disposition. Staff must also be informed immediately when the client is assessed as being a high risk for suicide in order to initiate appropriate observational interventions.

Suggested Reading

Antai-Otong, D (2003). Suicide: Life span considerations. *Nurisng Clinics of North America, 38,* 137–150.

Beck, AT (1991). *Cognitive Therapy and Emotional Disorders.* New York: International Universities Press.

Beck, JC & Baxter, P (1998). The violent patient. In Lifson, LE & Simon, RI (Eds.). *The Mental Health Practitioner and the Law: A Comprehensive Handbook* (pp. 153–165) Cambridge, MA: Harvard University Press.

Bostwick, J & Pankratz, AS (2000). Affective disorders and suicidal risk: A reexamination. *American Journal of Psychiatry, 157,* 1925–1932.

Denison, ME; Paredes, A & Boothm JB (1997). Alcohol and cocaine interactions and aggressive behaviors. In M Galanter (Ed.). *Recent Developments in Alcoholism, Vol 13. Alcoholism and Violence.* New York: Plenum.

Fawcett, J; Clark, DC; & Busch, KA (1993). Assessing and treating the patient at risk for suicide. *Psychiatric Annals, 23,* 244–255.

Harris, EC & Barraclough, B (1997). Suicide as an outcome for mental disorders: A meta-analysis. *British Journal of Psychiatry, 170,* 205–228.

Hornig, CD & McNally, RJ (1995). Panic disorder and suicide attempt: A reanalysis of data from the Epidemiologic Catchment Area study. *British Journal of Psychiatry, 167,* 76–79.

Hughes, DH (1996). Implications of recent court rulings for crisis and psychiatric emergency services. *Psychiatric Annals, 47,* 1332–1333.

Jacobs, DG (1999). *Guide to Suicide Assessment and Intervention.* San Francisco: Jossey-Bass.

Kessler, RC, Borges, G & Walters, EE (1999). Prevalence and risk factors for lifetime suicide attempts in the National Comorbidity Survey. *Archives of General Psychiatry, 56,* 617–626.

Kleepies, PM & Dettmer, E (2000). An evidenced-based approach to evaluating and managing suicidal emergencies. *Journal of Clinical Psychology, 59,* 1109–1130.

McCraig, LF & Strussman, BJ (1997). National hospital ambulatory care survey: 1996. In CDC. Emergency department summary: Advance data from Vital Statistics. No. 293. Hyattsville, MD: National Center for Health Statistics.

Motto, JA (1999). Critical points in the assessment and management of suicide risk. In DG Jacobs (Ed). *The Harvard Medical School Guide to Suicide Assessment and Intervention* (pp. 224–238). San Francisco: Jossey-Bass.

Peters, KD; Kochanek, KD & Murphy, SL (1998). Deaths: final data for 1996. In CDC. National vital statistics reports. Vol. 47, No. 9. Hyattsville, MD: National Center for Health Statistics.

Radomsky, ED; Haas, GL; Mann, JJ & Sweeney, JA (1999). Suicidal behavior in patients with schizophrenia and other psychotic disorders. *American Journal of Psychiatry, 156,* 1590–1595.

Simon, RI (1999). *Concise Guide to Psychiatric and the Law for Clinicians,* 2nd ed. Washington, DC: American Psychiatric Press.

Simon, RI & Goetz, S (1999). Forensic issues in the psychiatric emergency department. *Psychiatric Clinics of North America, 22,* 851–864.

Stack, S (1998a). The relationship between culture and suicide: An analysis of African Americans. *Transcultural Psychiatry, 35,* 253–269.

Stack, S (1998b). Education and risk of suicide: An analysis of African Americans. *Sociological Focus, 31,* 295–302.

Weiss, RD & Hufford, MR (1999). Substance abuse and suicide. DG Jacobs (Ed). *The Harvard Medical School Guide to Suicide Assessment and Intervention* (pp. 300–310). San Francisco: Jossey-Bass.

Risk Factors: Older Adults

Suicide among older white men is a critical health problem and reducing this high prevalence is a national priority. People 65 years and older have the highest rate of completed suicide at a rate of six times the rate of all ages combined (Centers for Disease Control and Prevention, 1997; McIntosh, 1995; Turvey, Conwell, Jones,Phillips, Simonsick et al, 2002). Data from these studies suggest the importance of assessing all age groups, particularly older adults who seldom talk about their distress and self harm ideations.

A significant number of older adults have firearms available in their homes (Oslin, Zubritsky, Brown, Mullaby, Puliafico et al, 2004). Of particular interest are the lethal methods older adults use to kill themselves. It is actually the higher lethality methods used by this age group that distinguishes suicide between the young and old. Firearms are the most common method of suicide among older adult men and women. Among older adults in extended care facilities, self-starvation may be suicidal although they deny that their behavior is self-destructive. The availability (e.g. unlocked gun cases, loaded guns) of firearms that also increases the risk of suicide in this age group. One study (Wintemute, Parham, Beaumont, Wright & Drake, 1999) found that the risk of suicide increased during the first year handguns were purchased further indicating inquiries about accessibility and purchase date.

Clinicians must carefully screen older adults and other age groups for firearm accessibility. In addition, they must also educate families and significant others about safe storage practices of firearms as a preventive measure among older adults presenting with depression or emotional distress and suicidal ideations.

Psychosocial factors contribute to the high rate of suicide in older adults. Older adults at risk of suicide are more likely to cite loneliness as a major reason for suicide along with other psychosocial stressors, such as financial concerns, depression, emotional distress, poor perceived health, physical impairment, alcohol problems, feelings of helplessness, hopelessness, inadequacy and isolation (Antai-Otong, 2003; Turvey, et al. 2002).

Most older adults who commit suicide suffer from medical and psychiatric illnesses. Studies show that more than 70 % of older adults who commit suicide have visited their physician within one month of their suicide, and a third within one week of their suicide. Furthermore, most of these clients presented with vague physical symptoms and denial of psychological distress (Conwell, Duberstein, Cox, et al, 1996; Conwell, 1997; Beautrais, 2002; Turvey, et al, 2002). Suicide in older adults is more likely to be planned than impulsive—suggesting that the clinician may be able to reduce its occurrence.

Clinical implications suggest that all older adults must be assessed for suicide, particularly when they have vague somatic complaints. Often these clients and their families incorrectly attribute depressive symptoms and suicidal ideations to growing old. Additionally, older adults are less likely to seek mental or psychiatric emergency services or endorse a depressed mood or suicidal ideations, particularly older men, hence they must be asked direct questions and informed that depression is a treatable illness.

General Considerations for Working with the Suicidal Older Adult

1. In addition to the previous discussion about suicide, it is imperative for *all* older men and women to be thoroughly assessed for suicide and homicide risk and provided immediate interventions to reduce suicide in this age group

2. Approach clients from an individual and culturally sensitive perspective. This also involves discerning the level of suicidality acceptability. Lower cultural approval of suicide often parallels lower suicide rates, particularly among Asian-Americans, Hispanic, or Latino-American and African-Americas

Disposition/Treatment

Disposition and treatment options have been previously discussed in this chapter. Older adults will also benefit from family crisis interventions and assertive outreach community services that target age-specific issues of older adults. Family members must also be educated about recurrent suicidal ideations and parameters for seeking emergency interventions.

Suggested Reading

Antai-Otong, D (2003). *Psychiatric Nursing: Biological and Behavioral Concepts.* Clifton Park, NY: Delmar Thomson Learning.

Centers for Disease Control and Prevention (1997). Available online: http://www.cdc.gov/ncipc/data/us9794/Suic.htm.

Conwell, Y (1997). Management of suicidal behavior in the elderly. *Psychiatric Clinics of North America, 20,* 667–683.

Conwell, Y; Duberstein, PR; Cox, C; Herrmann, JF; Forbes, NT, & Caine, ED. (1998). Age differences in behaviors leading to completed suicide. *American Journal of Geriatric Psychiatry, 6,* 122–126.

Conwell, Y; Duberstein, PR; Cox, C; et al, (1996). Relationship of age and Axis I diagnoses in victims of completed suicide: A psychological autopsy study. *American Journal of Psychiatry, 158,* 1001–1008.

McIntosh, JL (1995). Suicide prevention in the elderly (ages 65–99). *Suicide and Life-Threatening Behavior, 25,* 180–192.

Oslin, DW; Zubritsky, C; Brown, G; Mullahy, M; Puliafico, A & Have, TH (2004). Managing suicide risk in late life: Access to firearms as a public health risk. *American Journal of Geriatric Psychiatry, 12,* 30–36.

Pearson, JL (2000). Suicidal behavior in later life: Research update. In Maris, RW; Canetto, SS; McIntosh, JL & Silverman, MM (Eds.). *Review of Suicidology, 2000.* New York: Guilford Press.

The Gallup Organization (1992): *Executive Summary; Attitude and Incidence of Suicide Among the Elderly.* The Gallup Organization, Inc. Princeton, New Jersey.

Turvey, CL; Conwell, Y; Jones, MP; Phillips, C; Simonsick, E; Pearson, JL & Wallace, W (2002). Risk factors for late-life suicide: A prospective, community-based study. *American Journal of Geriatric Psychiatry, 10,* 398–406.

Uncapper, H & Arean, PA (2000). Physicians are less likely to treat suicidal ideation in older patients. *Journal of the American Geriatrics Society, 48,* 188–192.

Wintemute, GJ; Parham, CA; Beaumont, JJ; Wright & Drake, (1999). Mortality among recent purchasers of handguns. *New England Journal of Medicine, 341,* 1583–1589.

Risk Factors: Adolescents

The growing incidence of suicide and attempted suicide among today's youth is distressing. The prevalence of suicide and suicide attempts among children and adolescents suggests that clinicians must be able to identify risk factors and provide appropriate interventions. Prevention of suicide in youth has been a major health focus over the past decade. Major risk factors for suicide in adolescents include impaired social adjustment, stressful life events, mood and substance-related disorders. Of these factors the *strongest predictors* of child and adolescent suicide include *poor social adjustment* and the presence of a *mood disorder* prior to the suicide attempt (Pfeffer, et al, 1993).

In the assessment of suicidal ideation and behavior, clinicians must establish the presence and degree of suicidal intent or lethality. Assessing the degree of suicidal intent involves discerning a balance between the wish to die and live. In children, like adults, suicide intent often parallels a sense of hopelessness. Direct clinical observation of children suggests that their level of understanding about the potential lethality of suicidal behaviors varies. For instance, a 6-year-old child may wish to die and ingest two vitamins and believe that they are lethal. Assessing suicide intent in children requires an understanding of the potential lethality of a suicide attempt, actual lethality of an act, and motives for suicidal behavior. Children's conceptualization of death exists on a cognitive-developmental continuum and influences their perception about suicide. In essence, clinicians working with children and adolescents presenting with suicidal thoughts, intent, and/or a wish to die must also appreciate their developmental and cognitive grasp of this behavior. They must also recognize developmental factors that impact their verbal skills, finality of death and reliability.

Information about the youth's level of lethality and ability to understand suicidal behavior, intent and motivation also requires gathering information from parents or primary caregivers. Data collections from several sources also provide information about similarities and discrepancies about the child's suicidal ideation and behavior. Interviewing children and their parents can be challenging, especially in the context of parental or family dysfunction. Parents offer important information about the child, particularly their observations, change in behavior and mood and an accurate depiction of the child's symptoms.

Major considerations for assessing the suicidal child/adolescent include providing an emotionally and safe environment. Any child/youth who expresses suicidal ideations must be taken just as serious as an adult who actually attempts suicide. Age-specific interviewing skills and treatment are essential in creating a safe environment and quality mental health care for the suicidal youth.

General Considerations for the Suicidal Adolescent and Family

Interviewing youth and their parents is very stressful and challenging. Clinicians must allow for ample time when working with children and their parents. The following format is useful in eliciting information from the child and parents.

1. Interview the child/adolescent alone

   • assess for suicidal ideations, motivation, and intent
   • identify the presenting problem—family or personal stressors

   Are you thinking about killing yourself? If so, how?

   Did you ever feel so sad or upset that you did not want to live?

   Have you ever done anything dangerous that you knew was harmful?

   Have you ever thought about or tried to kill yourself?

   After you tried to kill yourself did you still want to die, or want to live?

   How often do you think about killing yourself?

   Have any of your friends or acquaintances/relatives killed him or herself?

   • Discern the status of the youth's relationship with parents and peers, and use of free time
   • Assess child/adolescent's perception of the present visit to psychiatric emergency
   • Ask about suicidal ideations, gestures and means, including access to weapons or other dangerous items, and past attempts
   • Perform an age-specific mental status examination-children and adolescents are likely to complain of being irritable.
   • Assess eating habits, sleeping patterns, friends, and present stressors than sad or depressed

47

- Assess the youth's understanding about the finality of death
- Assess for mental illness, including mood, anxiety, psychosis, and substance use/abuse
- Consider immediate hospitalization when the child is deemed to be an imminent danger to self and/or others
- Ask requests to determine the youth's outlook on life, self-esteem, and sense of hope

2. Interview the parent(s) alone

- Ask about their concerns or reasons for bringing the child
- Assess present stressful life events (particularly those that threaten family integrity)
- Assess the parent's perception of the present family crisis
- Discern family history of mental illness, suicide attempts, mood and substance-related disorders
- Assess the parents' mental status
- Encourage parents to express their feelings and concerns about their child
- Inquire about child's present friendships, and home and academic performances
- Assess parents' ability to care for the child
- Assess their response to the youth's ideations, attempts and level of empathy
- Assess the nature of the marital or couple dyad
- Evaluate the family's coping and problem solving skills

3. Interview the child/adolescent with parents and assess

- the nature of the parent-child relationship
- present stressful life events

- role of cultural factors and ability to cope
- quality of family support systems and resources
- the role of the youth's symptoms on maintaining the family
- provision of family crisis therapy when indicated

Disposition and Treatment

Managing psychiatric emergencies with this age group requires a thorough evaluation of the child and parents or primary caregivers. Criteria for hospitalization are the same as for adults. When parents opt to monitor the child's behavior they sort out ways to watch the suicidal client and construct a schedule for taking turns. Other considerations for disposition include family crisis intervention, couples or family therapy.

Suggested Readings

Antai-Otong, D (2003). *Psychiatric Nursing: Biological and behavioral concepts.* Clifton Park, NY: Delmar Thomson Learning.

Beautrais, AL (2003). Suicide and serious suicide attempts in youth; A multiple-group comparison study. *American Journal of Psychiatry, 160,* 1093–1099.

Gould, MS; Fisher, P; Parides, M; Flory. M & Shaffer, D (1996). Psychosocial risk factors of child and adolescent completed suicide. *Archives of Psychiatry, 53,* 1155–1162.

Jacobsen, LK; Rabinowitz, I; Popper, MS; Solomon, RJ; Sokol, MS & Pffefer, CS (1994). Interviewing prepubertal children about suicidal ideation and behavior. *Journal of the American Academy of Child and Adolescent Psychiatry, 33,* 439–452.

Nock, MK & Kazdin, AE (2002). Examinations of affective, cognitive and behavioral factors and suicide-related outcomes in children and young adolescents. *Journal of Clinical Child and Adolescent Psychology, 31*, 48–58.

Parsons, C (2003). Caring for adolescents and families in crisis. *Nursing Clinics of North America, 38*, 111–122.

Pfeffer, CR; Klerman, GL; Hurt, SW; Kakuma, T; Peskin, JR; Siefker, CA (1993). Suicidal children grow up: Rates and psychological risk factors for suicide attempts during follow-up. *Journal of the Academy of Child and Adolescent Psychiatry, 32*, 106–113.

Pilowsky, DJ; Wu, LT & Anthony, JC (1999). Panic attacks and suicide attempts in mid-adolescence. *American Journal of Psychiatry, 156*, 1545–1549.

Wagner, KD; Rouleau, M & Joiner, T (2000). Cognitive factors related to suicidal ideation and resolution in psychiatrically hospitalized children and adolescents. *American Journal of Psychiatry, 157*, 2017–2021.

Schizophrenia and Other Psychotic Disorders

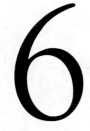

Epidemiology and Prevalence

1. The prevalence of schizophrenia remains 1% in the general population, culture and social class. The etiology of schizophrenia includes a genetic component and theories suggest that pathophysiological factors include an overactivity of dopamine in the mesolimbic system resulting in acute psychosis.

2. Other pathophysiological factors include structural abnormalities of the temporal lobe and limbic system encompassing the frontal lone to the inferior parietal cortex.

3. Antipsychotic agents are the primary agents used to treat schizophrenia and other psychotic disorders.

4. Acute psychosis and adverse drug reactions are the primary reasons for seeking psychiatric emergency services.

Evaluation

1. A client presenting with acute psychosis-out of touch with reality, is often responding to auditory or visual hallucinations, and because of delusions perceives clinicians as threatening.

2. Hallucinations and delusions in these clients are potentially life threatening and must be quickly assessed and treated. Clinicians must assess the nature of hallucinations including the presence of command hallucinations and focus on the following:

   • Whether hallucinations are suggestive of violence towards self or others

   • Presence of delusions or other beliefs that are consistent with hallucinations

   • The voices and their familiarity and whether the client has responded to them in the past

3. Command hallucinations are considered a risk factor for violence

4. The immediate control of dangerous or life-threatening behavior occurs as the clinician rules out medical conditions, such as delirium.

Differential Diagnosis

• Rule out medical conditions, such as delirium, drug toxicity, substance-related psychosis

• Rule out other psychiatric disorders, such as affective psychosis, such as bipolar disorder.

Acute Psychosis-Schizophrenia

A brief mental status examination and focused physical examination are critical assessment tools during the initial contact with the acutely psychotic client. Symptoms of schizophrenic psychosis are more likely to be more florid and bizarre than other psychotic disorders. Hallucinations in these clients tend to be in the third person ("Jennifer is evil") rather than the second person ("You are evil"). These clients are also more likely to experience auditory hallucinations that involve several voices—sometimes arguing about the client. (*See* **Table IV.**). Delusions in clients with schizophrenia are likely to be paranoid, grandiose, or disorganized.

Emergency management of psychosis begins with making an accurate differential diagnosis and subsequently implementing crisis management and initiating appropriate psychosocial and pharmacological interventions. Psychosocial interventions include approaching the client in a non-threatening, calm, yet firm manner. Firm verbal de-escalation is an important part of this process and involves using assertive communication to convey concern and care, yet expectations regarding this behavior. Clients experiencing acute psychosis are usually agitated, irritable and sensitive to environmental stimuli. Efforts to reduce environmental stimuli include using a normal tone voice and a quiet area, and ensuring staff safety. Staff safety involves making sure that properly trained help can be made available when needed and the client understands that efforts are available to control the situation. Calling the client by name and informing him or her that the staff is there to help regain a sense of control and offering medications will allay anxiety and reduce psychotic symptoms. (*See* **Table V.**)

Prior to medicating the client the clinician should be clear about the target symptoms—hallucinations and delusions, anxiety and agitation. It is critical that staff rule out major medical conditions that mimic psychiatric disorders because psychotropic agents can obscure the differential diagnosis and prolong the assessment process and initiation of appropriate interventions. Once the diagnosis of a psychiatric disorder is deter-

Table IV: Major Features of Acute Psychosis

Psychotic disorders: schizophrenia, schizoaffective disorder (see mood disorder for mood-related symptoms)

- hallucinations
- delusions
- thought disorganization
- bizarre behaviors
- flat or blunted affect (schizophrenia)

- loose associations
- perseveration
- social aloofness (schizophrenia)
- disoganized speech
- catatonic behavior-motoric immobility or stupor

Mood disorders, such as bipolar and major depression, with psychotic features, or schizoaffective disorder*

- hallucinations
- delusions
- thought disorganization
- rapid or pressured speech
- agitated, elated, or irritable mood

- racing thoughts
- flight of ideas
- circumstantiality
- tangentiality
- intrusiveness

Substance or general medical conditions*

(Same as above, but in each the disturbance stems from the direct effects of a substance (e.g. illicit or licit drugs) or a general medical condition (e.g. diabetes or hyperthyroidism). A diagnosis of a *general medical condition* requires an accurate differential diagnosis that guides the clinician's decision to initiate specific interventions. Normally, this involves correcting the underlying medical condition and providing reassurance and emotional support.

* requires a differential diagnosis

mined appropriate pharmacological interventions can be initiated. If the client's symptoms are deemed a medical conditions, such as fluid and electrolyte imbalance or urinary tract infection, appropriate medical consultations and referrals must be made. (*See* **Table VI.**)

Because the client presenting with acute psychosis experiences intense anxiety and agitation, efforts to reduce anxiety with a benzodiazepine also reduce psychosis and reduces the incidence of violence. Acute psychosis is generally treated with a combination of a neuroleptic, such as haloperidol (a high-potency agent) and a benzodiazepine, such as lorazepam (a short-acting agent) because they provide immediate con-

Table V: Psychosocial Interventions for Acute Psychosis

1. Support reality
2. Call client by name
3. Introduce self and acknowledge the client's distress
4. Use active listening skills and tell the client what you want to do and what you do not understand
5. Assess for the nature of hallucinations and delusions
6. Assess the client's level of dangerousness to self and/others
7. Do not approach an openly hostile client alone-get assistance
8. Afford a comfortable space between self and client (leg's length)
9. Do not touch or make sudden movements
10. Be aware of your personal feelings and behaviors

Table VI: Common Medical Conditions Associated with Secondary Psychosis

Medical Conditions	Medications
Endocrine • hyperthyroidism • postpartum mania **Metabolic** • hemodialysis • post operative state • Vitamin deficiences—B_{12}, folate, niacin, thiamine • cerebral hypoxia **Infection** • influenza • HIV • neurosyphillis **Neurologic** • vascular disease, stroke • traumatic brain injury	**Drugs** • cimetidine (Tagamet) • levo dopa • disulfiram (Antabuse) • BDZs—alprazolam (Xanax) • NSAIDS—ibuprofen (Motrin), naprosyn (Alleve) • cyproheptadine (Persantin) • thyroxine (thyroid replacement hormone) • corticosteroids • amphetamines • cimetidine • opiates and opioids • amantadine • bupropion • buspirone • folic acid • tricyclic antidepressants **Drug withdrawal** • Beta blockers (i.e., propanolol [Inderal])

trol. Some researchers believe that lorazepam alone or a combination of these two agents has been shown to be equally effective in treating psychotic agitation. This is questionable because even if the client's agitation abates, core psychotic symptoms remain—suggesting that a combination is more effective (Foster et al, 1997; Lenox, et al, 1992; Saltzman, et al, 1991). A major advantage of haloperidol is that it can be given by injection, unlike other neuroleptic agents, it is relatively safe and rapidly effective. A disadvantage of this medication is its side effect profile, including extrapyramidal side effects (EPS). Haloperidol should not be given to clients who have a history of neuroleptic malignant syndrome. Alternative treatment to the traditional haloperidol and lorazepam are the new atypical antipsychotic agents. Studies show that these medications have proven efficacy in the management of acute psychotic agitation and produce fewer EPS side effects than typical agents (Currier, Chou, Feifel, Bossie, Turkoz, et al, 2004; Heck, Haffmans, de Groot, & Hoencamp, 2000) (*See* **Table VII.**)

Because of fewer clients being hospitalized and shorter lengths of stay, the increase of acutely psychotic clients presenting in the ED is on the rise. An increase in these clients in the ED compels clinicians to use astute observational and clinical skills to quickly assess psychotic symptoms and make differential diagnoses.

Acute Psychosis: Schizoaffective Disorder

Clients presenting with schizoaffective disorder have symptoms consistent with schizophrenia with prominent mood disturbances, such as depressed, manic or mixed. An accurate diagnosis of this disorder requires a thorough psychiatric history. The primary basis to the diagnosis, is a history of psychosis in the absence of mood symptoms, which is often very challenging to the clinician in the ED.

Table VII: The Management of Acute Psychosis

Specific Psychotic Disorder	Legal Considerations: Pharmacological Interventions	Side Effects

Schizophrenia and other psychotic disorders	**Legal Considerations**
	
	1. Assess the client's ability to participate in the decision about medication
	2. Consider past treatment responses and adverse drug reactions
	
	Pharmacological Interventions
	
	1. Rapid tranquilization is normally a safe and effective approach that controls agitation, anxiety, tension, or excitement in potentially violent clients.
	2. This can be accomplished by an intramuscular injection (IM) or oral concentrate antipsychotic such as
	  • haloperidol 2-4 mg* over 30-60 minutes (unless the client has a history of neuroleptic malignant syndrome)
	  • lorazepam (1-2 mg IM/po to enhance the reduce anxiety and agitation and enhance the effects of neuroleptic)
	
	* lower dose for clients ≥ 65 years of age
		Extrapyrimadal Side Effects (EPS)
		
		a. **Dystonias** (prolonged and involuntary muscular contractions, facial grimacing, throat tightness, and posturing of neck, back or trunk)—can be life-threatening if it produces laryngeal dystonia *or affects muscle related to breathing (occurs 1-2 hours after first dose of neuroleptic)*
		
		b. **Parkinsonism**—triad of course tremor, muscular rigidity, and bradykinesia (masklike facies or difficulty initiating movements) *(occurs after 2-3 months of treatment)*
		
		c. **Akathesia**—client's subjective complaint of restlessness, and observable pacing and rocking *(occurs during early treatment of increase in dose of neuroleptic)*
		
		d. **Neuroleptic malignant syndome (NMS)**—severe muscle rigidity, high fever, altered mental status,and autonomic instability (high mortality rate and requires immediate medical intervention)

Table VII: The Management of Acute Psychosis *(Continued)*

Specific Psychotic Disorder	Legal Considerations: Pharmacological Interventions	Side Effects
		Note: EPS and NMS are likely to be associated with high potency agents, such as haloperidol and less with atypical neuroleptics. They are also dose-related. **Treatment includes:** reduce dose or switch to atypical agent, and administer • anticholinergic and antihistamine agents: IM/po: • benztropine 1–2 mg or diphenhydramine 25–50 mg (repeat within 30 min PRN), which usually reduce reactions within 1–2

Treatment of acute psychotic symptoms in these clients is the same as acute schizophrenic symptoms except a combination of mood stabilizer (bipolar-manic symptoms) or antidepressant (depression) is added to manage mood disturbances.

Substance-Induced Psychosis

Psychiatric emergency management of substance-induced psychosis is similar to the treatment of schizophrenia. Establishing a safe and calm environment is critical for dealing with the client who has intense paranoia and impulsivity. When the client has problems maintaining control, efforts to establish control through physical restraints or containment are essential until pharmacological interventions allay anxiety and produce their calming effects. (*See* **Table VIII.**) Pharmacological agents used to manage these symptoms include short acting benzodiazepines, such as lorazepam and psychosocial interventions. A combination of droperidol (a low-potency neuroleptic) and lorazepam are uniquely safe for the management of acute substance-related psychosis and agitation.

Table VIII: Pharmacological Management: Stimulant-Induced Psychosis

- Low-dose antipsychotic and lorazepam (2–5 mg IM or IV)
- Antipsychotic useful in the treatment of stimulant induced psychosis 1–2 doses every 30–60 minute interval produces rapid and prolonged sedation
- Monitor vital signs and assess for desired and adverse drug reactions

Suggested Readings

American Psychiatric Association (2000). Diagnostic and statistical manual of mental disorders, 4th edition, text revision. Washington, DC: American Psychiatric Association.

Antai-Otong, D (2004). Pharmacologic and psychosocial considerations in the management of schizophrenia. CME offering. *Federal Practitioner, 21,* 89–102.

Antai-Otong, D (2003). *Psychiatric Nursing: Biological and behavioral concepts.* Clifton Park, NY: Delmar Thomson Learning.

Bieniek, SA; Ownby, RL; Penalver, J; et al (1998). A double-blind study of lorazepam versus the combination of haloperidol and lorazepam in managing agitation. *Pharmacotherapy, 18,* 57–62.

Chambers, RA & Druss, BG (1999). Droperidal: Efficacy and side effects in psychiatric emergencies. *Journal of Clinical Psychiatry, 60,* 664–667.

Currier, GW; Chou, JC; Feifel, D; Bossie, CA; Turkoz, I; Mahmoud, RA; Gharabawi, GM (2004). Acute management of psychotic agitation: A randomized comparison of oral treatment with risperidone and lorazepam versus intramuscular treatment with haloperidol and lorazepam. *Journal of Clinical Psychiatry, 65,* 386–394.

Foster, S; Kessek, J; Berman, ME & Simpson, GM (1997). Efficacy of lorazepam and haloperidol for rapid tranquilization in a psychiatric emergency room setting. *International Clinical Psychopharmacology, 12,* 175–179.

Heck, AH; Haffmans, PMJ; de Groot, IW & Hoencamp, E (2000). Risperidone versus haloperidol in psychotic patients with disturbing antipsychotic-induced extrapyramidal symptoms: A double-blind, multi-center trial. *Schizophrenia Research, 46,* 97–105.

Hilliard, JR (1998). Emergency treatment of acute psychosis. *Journal of Clinical Psychiatry, 59 (suppl 1),* 57–60.

Geriatric Emergencies

7

Epidemiology and Prevalence

1. As the population ages, there will be a greater need for clinicians to recognize complex symptoms of dementia and other cognitive disorders in the older population.

2. Delirium and dementia are seen comorbidly in about 30% to 60% of older adults in general hospital settings (Marcantonio, Flacker, Wright, & Resnick, 2001; Webster & Holroyd, 2000). These conditions also are associated with increased length of stays, higher hospital costs and greater likelihood of nursing home placement at discharge (Saravay, Kaplowitz, Kurek, Zeman, Pollack, et al, 2004).

3. Age specific changes stemming from brain changes, pharmocokinetic and pharmocodynamic changes increase the risk of cognitive disturbances in older adults. Predictably, comorbid physical illnesses, social isolation, sensory deficits, polypharmacy, and substance-related disorders are also likely to increase the prevalence of dementia and delirium.

Evaluation

Older adults are often embarrassed or hesitant about seeking psychiatric treatment and are likely to be referred for evaluation from various health care providers. Referrals are likely to be made after medical conditions have been ruled out or by extended care facilities and/or concerned family members because of mental status changes. When making a differential diagnosis of geriatric emergencies it is imperative for clinicians to distinguish between age-related changes and other medical and psychiatric conditions.

Clinicians working with older adults must approach them calmly and in a timely manner to manage the problem and prevent escalation. Major symptoms seen in this age group include cognitive disturbances-memory problems, confusion-agitation, combativeness, and inability to participate in treatment decisions. A numbers of factors increase the risk of psychiatric emergencies in older adults and they include polypharmacy, depression, abuse and neglect and exacerbation of psychiatric illnesses. Of particular interest to clinicians working with older adults is the high incidence of delirium produced by most psychotropic medications, including lithium, other mood stabilizers, antidepressants including tricyclic antidepressants (i.e., amitryptiline [Elavil]), selective serotonin reuptake inhibitors (i.e., fluoxetine [Prozac]) and benzodiazepines (i.e., diazepam [Valium]). Management of these symptoms is complex because they are similar to those found in other medical conditions including endocrine disorders and dementia, psychiatric disorders, and substance-related disorders.

The initial aspect of managing a geriatric emergency is making an accurate differential diagnosis. Clinicians need to determine the most likely underlying medical condition and evaluate its functional effects. Because many of these emergencies are linked to underlying medical conditions, such as endocrine disorders, B_{12} deficiency, and polypharmacy, an in-depth physical examination that includes laboratory and other diagnostic test must be performed.

1. *History taking* should focus on the specific cognitive and behavioral changes in the client, their evolution over time, and symptoms linking them to medical, neurologic, or psychiatric conditions. A thorough history should include:

   • A *review of prescription and non prescription drugs* that interfere with cognitive function, such as antihypertensive agents, anticholinergic agents (i.e., diphenhydramine [Benadryl]), sedative-hynoptics.
   • Recent head trauma or falls
   • History of surgery, anesthesia
   • Data from significant others regarding the client's functional status, history of delirium or dementia, depression, or stroke

2. *Mental status screening* should comprise an assessment to rule out depression and cognitive disorders. Standardized instruments such as the Mini Mental Status Examination offer clinicians another way to assist in making a differential diagnosis. Areas of particular interest during the psychiatric assessment include:

   • Cognition
   • Mood disorders (i.e., major depressive episode, bipolar disorder, Type I)—memory impairment, concentration difficulties, and reduction in intellectual abilities
   • Psychosis
   • Level of dangerousness to self and others
   • Abuse or neglect

3. *Medical evaluations* must include data from the psychosocial assessment and consist of a complete physical examination, laboratory and diagnostic studies such as a blood chemistry panel,

complete blood count, thyroid panel, Vitamin B_{12}, folate and thiamine levels, and screening for infectious diseases.

A. Delirium: A Medical Emergency

1. Delirium is one of the most misdiagnosed medical conditions in older adults. The exact cause of delirium is poorly understood. It has an acute onset and is characterized by changes in cognition and consciousness. Although the onset is acute, manifestations may be transitory and persist for days or months.

2. This potentially reversible medical disorder often arises from an underlying medical condition or drug toxicity that disrupts cerebral metabolism and regulation of biochemical processes. There are many conditions that cause delirium-infections, metabolic disorders, fluid and electrolyte imbalance, alcohol withdrawal and polypharmacy. These factors are believed to disrupt brain metabolism and neurochemical reactions.

3. Other factors that increase the risk of delirium include age over 80 years, fractures during hospital stays, male gender, urinary retention, and fecal impaction. (*See* **Table IX.**)

4. Delirium often develops rapidly in older clients with an acute illness or injury.

Differential Diagnosis

Early recognition of delirium is important because of increased mortality and morbidity. Efforts to identify the underlying medical condition or drug toxicity are imperative to resolve the delirium and reduce death. These clients must be referred for immediate medical evaluation and treatment.

Table IX: Common Medical Conditions that Cause Delirium

Infections

Endocrine disorders
- pancreas
- thyroid
- parathyroid
- pituitary

Nutritional or vitamin deficiencies
- malnutrition
- fluid and electrolyte imbalance
- folate, vitamin B_{12} and thiamine deficiencies
- constipation

Diseases of major organs
- liver
- kidney
- cardiovascular, including arrythymias and anemia
- neurological
- lung, including hypoxia

Drugs and poisons
- anticholinergic agents, such as diphenhydramine (Benadryl)
- heavy metals, such as lead
- antihypertensive agents
- histamine antagonists, such as cimetidine (Tagamet)
- cardiac glycosides
- opioid analgesics
- sedatives, including alcohol, benzodiazepines and hynotics
- steroids
- antidepressants including SSRIs and tertiary amines, such as imipramine
- anticonvulsants
- antipsychotic or neuroleptic agents

Differential diagnosis can be determined by information gathered from the bio-psychosocial examinations—history, duration and course of symptoms and duration and timing of functional decline. Additional information includes the results from the physical exam, MSE, and diagnostic studies.

Physical Examination

- abnormal vital signs
- fluctuation in blood pressure
- elevated temperature
- tachycardia—increased heart rate
- increased respirations
- headaches
- nystagmus
- motor disturbances—ataxia, hyperreflexia, tremors
- dilated pupils
- flushing, dry skin
- fluctuating consciousness
- lethargy
- diaphoresis (sweating) or dry skin
- abnormal laboratory findings (depend upon underlying medical condition)

Mental Status Examination

Characteristic symptoms of delirium include:

- an acute, reversible state of confusion or *cloudiness of sensorium*—hallmark of delirium
- *fluctuating symptoms—alternating with lucid periods*
- symptoms may fluctuate and persist for days or months
- a disturbance in consciousness and change in cognition that develops over a short duration and fluctuates over the course of the day
- frequently unrecognized or misdiagnosed in older adults
- *disorientation*—time and place, but rarely to person
- *inability to focus or sustain attention*

- *agitation*
- *memory impairment*—short and long term memory disturbances
- perceptual disturbances—*usually visual hallucinations*—colorful, vivid and well defined as well as illusions and delusions
- psychomotor changes
- personality changes
- labile mood, anxiety or disruptive/combative behavior
- symptoms may be more pronounced in the evening ("sun-downing")

Management

Psychosocial Interventions

Although psychosocial interventions alone cannot treat delirium they help to reduce the client's anxiety and agitation. It is important for the clinician to reduce environmental stimuli by reducing noises, bright lights and number of interpersonal contacts. Approach the client in a calm non-threatening manner and use direct and clear statements. Ensuring safety also means making sure that someone remains with the client at all times and that the client is reoriented as needed. Make sure that the bed is in its lowest position and that a means of restraining the client, if necessary, is available. Using restraints should be the last resort for dealing with a delirious combative client. Remind family members that delirium is usually reversible and improves over time.

Additional psychosocial interventions include close assessment of the clients mental and physical status (i.e., vital and neurological signs). These data provide important information about changes in the client's condition. Assess the client's self-care needs and offer assistance to maintain emotional and physical integrity. Anticipate the client's anxiety and intervene appropriately using a calm and reassuring approach and initiating pharmacological interventions as indicated.

Pharmacological Interventions

The mere presence of delirium is not an indication for pharmacological intervention. The need for this approach must be clearly identified, documented, and continually reassessed. Clinical implications for pharmacological interventions include assaultive and combative behaviors. Given the likelihood of comorbid medical conditions and concomitant medications, pharmacological interventions may be needed to manage common behavioral disturbances that often result in psychotic symptoms. A thorough medical evaluation to discern the underlying medical condition is imperative prior to initiating pharmacological agents.

Major pharmacological interventions include low dose benzodiazepines and neuroleptic medications—both typical (i.e., haloperidol) and atypical (quetiapine). High-potency neuroleptics, such as haloperidol, are preferred because they have fewer anticholinergic side effects (these can worsen delirium) and minimal hypotensive effects. Major disadvantages of haloperidol include extrapyramidal side effects (EPS) and the potential to actually prolong delirium and increase the risk of producing stupor. Recommended doses for older adults with mild delirium is 0.25–0.5 mg orally or 0.125 mg–0.25 mg IM (Flacker & Marcantonio, 1998). Clients receiving this medication must be constantly assessed for desired and adverse drug reactions.

Overall treatment of the delirious client involves treating the primary condition leading to delirium, removing contributing factors (i.e., metabolic, physiologic, pharmacologic) and supporting the client and their family.

Disposition

Consult with medical staff regarding this medical emergency. Most delirious clients are hospitalized for further evaluation and treatment.

If the client has transitory symptoms and is medically and psychiatrically stable, the client may be discharged to the family and given instructions regarding his or her care and follow up appointment.

B. Dementia

1. It is projected that up to 90% of clients with dementia will develop considerable behavioral problems over their lifetime. (Mega, et. al, 1996; Tariot, 1999)

2. Dementia is a major and increasing health problem. A major problem for clients with dementa and their caregivers is the noncognitive mental and behavioral disturbances. Understandably, the most serious disturbance is physical aggression or violent behavior. Over time these behaviors cause injury, mental distress and suffering and increase the risk of elder abuse.

3. Dementia is a general term for a chronic and progressive disorder of mental or cognitive function that produces a loss of intellectual and other higher brain functions. Almost half of people with dementia have a treatable or reversible form. Most people associate dementia with Alzheimer's disease, which often generates pessimism in clinicians. Dementia alone is not necessarily associated with a psychiatric emergency; however, many of these clients are brought in by caregivers or concerned friends because of behavioral and mental manifestations of an underlying dementia.

4. If the client is disoriented he or she is probably incompetent. Depending on the client's mental status and ability to make informed consent decisions or competence, clinicians must obtain consent from family members or caregivers or legal guardian until the crisis situation is resolved.

Differential Diagnosis

1. The goal of clinicians when these clients present exhibiting disruptive or aggressive behaviors and mental status changes is making a differential diagnosis and affording the client safe and appropriate treatment. Of particular importance is for clinicians to make a rapid diagnosis of reversible dementias. Rapid differential diagnosis enables clinicians to initiate interventions that correct the underlying medical condition and deter its deleterious course and prevent permanent pathological changes in the brain.

2. Dementia may be due to any of the following medical conditions:

   - Parkinson's disease*
   - Cerebrovascular disease*
   - Alzheimer's disease*
   - Medications
   - Depression
   - Metabolic deficiencies
   - Nutritional deficiencies
   - Huntington's disease*
   - Hypothyroidism
   - Brain tumor
   - B_{12} deficiency

   * irreversible dementias

3. Criteria for diagnosis of dementia include data that are collected from the client, observation and MSE, and caregivers. Asking questions that elicit history of symptoms, changes in memory, and functional status enable clinicians to explore the

course, onset, and reasons for present visit. Family members may also exhibit symptoms of depression or major medical problems stemming from caring for their loved one.

4. Assessing their level of functioning and ability to care for the client is just as relevant as the client's mental and physical assessment. This data provides a basis for the client's disposition and referral, particularly if the caregiver is unable to care for the client.

    A. *Mental Status Examination*

    - Impaired memory
    - Impaired cognitive function–language, spatial ability, reasoning, abstraction, and judgment
    - Clear sensorium
    - Personality or behavioral changes (*See* **Table X.**)

The client with an *irreversible dementia*, such as AD, may present with mild, moderate or severe symptoms. Symptoms of AD generally consist of an insidious and gradual-progressive course.

1. Additionally, these clients have problems with recent and remote memory deficits, use poor judgement and have difficulty with math and problem solving. Information obtained from family members or caregivers about the client's daily routine is invaluable, particularly if the client insists on driving.

2. Family members may also report that their loved one has been getting lost and has been brought home by local law officers. They may also report that the client has problems balancing the checkbook, performing basic self-care activities, including bathing or buttoning their clothes.

3. During the middle and latter stages of AD, these clients have problems naming common objects (anomia), such as a watch

Table X: Stages of Alzheimer's Disease

Stage I

- forgetfulness
- alert and oriented
- memory impairment
- disorientation
- restlessness
- anxiety
- shortened attention span
- some insight and awareness of condition expressed
- depression
- compensates forgetfulness by using notes or lists
- poor acquisition of new information
- personality changes

Stage II

- marked memory loss
- disorientation
- gets lost easily and attributes forgetfulness to "old age"
- denial
- confabulation
- self care deficits
- begins to experience global decline
- wandering behaviors increase with severity of cognitive deficits
- apathy and social aloofness
- agnosia (difficulty interpreting sensory stimuli)
- aphasis (difficulty generating speech)
- apraxia (inability to organize motor functioning)
- anomia (inability to name objects)

Stage III

- complete loss of ability to care for self
- social withdrawal
- judgement and decision making greatly impaired
- marked confusion
- spends most of time in bed or chair
- no longer recognize loved ones
- difficulty swallowing/eating
- death often results from medical complications, such as pneumonia, decubiti, and urinary tract infections

or pencil; recognizing family members (agnosia); difficulty carrying out motor function (apraxia), such as lacing their shoes; and language difficulties (aphasia).

4. It is imperative for the clinician to get a sense of duration and course of symptoms and work with other health care professionals to establish a diagnosis.

The family also reports a *history of progressive behavioral disturbances,* such as fighting, cursing, hitting or disrobing inappropriately. Understanding the basis of these behaviors enables the clinician to educate family members about the disease and reduce elder abuse. Clients with high dependency needs are likely to become victims of elder abuse. During the mental status examination the clinician must also observe the family's interactions with the client and convey empathy.

B. *Physical Examinations* involves a thorough physical examination and ordering of appropriate laboratory and diagnostic studies to discern the basis of the client's present symptoms.

Management of Disruptive or Aggressive Behavior

Psychosocial and Pharmacological Interventions

Table XI: Management of Disruptive or Aggressive Behaviors in Alzheimer's Disease

Behavior	Psychosocial Interventions	Pharmacological Interventions
suspiciousness, paranoia, agitation	• well lit room • moderate stimulation • familiar objects in view	low dose antipsychotic agent and short acting benzodiazepine

Table XI: Management of Disruptive or Aggressive Behaviors in Alzheimer's Disease (Continued)

Behavior	Psychosocial Interventions	Pharmacological Interventions
wandering, pacing	• structured activities • secure locks/doors • planned daily activities • placing lines on the floor	
hitting, agitation, aggressiveness	• avoid activities that precipitate behavior • reduce stimuli • distract patient	low dose antipsychotic agent and short acting benzodiazepine
yelling, shouting, cursing	• identify source of pain, if cause • touch therapy • music therapy • environmental stimuli • avoiding restraints	trazodone, buspirone, SSRIs, depakote

Disposition

Consult with medical staff and referral is based on the client's medical and psychiatric status. These clients are most likely to be hospitalized for further evaluation to discern underlying cause of dementia and treatment of behavioral symptoms. Clinicians must also educate caregivers and make appropriate community referrals, including respite care.

Suggested Reading

American Psychiatric Association (1997). Practice guideline for the treatment of patients with Alzheimer's diesease and other dementias in late life. *American Journal of Psychiatry, 154* (Suppl), 1–39.

Antai-Otong, D (2003). Managing geriatric psychiatric emergencies: Delirium and dementia. *Nursing Clinics of North America, 38,* 123–135.

Blazer, D (1998). Geriatric psychiatry matures: Advantages and problems as the psychiatry of old grows older. *Current Opinion in Psychiatry, 11,* 401–403.

Blazer, DG (2000). Psychiatry and the oldest old. *American Journal of Psychiatry, 157,* 1915–1924.

Chan, D & Brennan, NJ (1999). Delirium: Making the diagnosis, improving the prognosis. *Geriatrics, 54,* 28–42.

Dyck, G (1997). Management of geriatric behavior problems. *Psychiatric Clinics of North America, 20,* 165–180.

Flacker, JM & Marcantonio, ER (1998). Delirium in the elderly. *Drugs & Aging, 13,* 119–130.

Jacobson, DA (1997). Delirium in the elderly. *Psychiatric Clinics of North America, 20,* 91–110.

Levkoff, SE; Evans, DA; Liptzin, B; Wetle, T; Reilly, C; Pilgrim, D; Schor, J & Rowe, J (1992). Delirium: The occurrence and persistence of symptoms among elderly hospitalized patients. *Archives of Internal Medicine, 152,* 334–340.

Marcantonio, ER; Flacker, JM; Wright, RJ & Resnick, NM (2000). Reducing delirium after hip fracture: A randomized trial. *Journal of the American Geriatric Society, 49,* 516–522.

Mega, MS; Cummings, JL; Fiorella, T & Gornbein, J (1996). The spectrum of behavioral change in Alzheimer's disease. *Neurology, 46,* 130–135.

Targum, SD & Abbott, JL (1999). Psychoses in the elderly: A spectrum of disorders. *Journal of Clinical Psychiatry, 60 (suppl 8),* 4–10.

Saravay, SM; Kaplowitz, M; Kurek, J; Zeman, D; Pollack, S; et al, (2004). How do delirium and dementia increase length of stay of elderly general medical inpatients. *Psychosomatics, 45,* 235–242.

Tariot, PN (1999). Treatment of agitation in dementia. *Journal of Clinical Psychiatry, 60 (suppl 8),* 11–20.

Webster, R & Holyroyd, S (2001). Prevalence of psychotic symptoms in delirium. *Psychosomatics, 41,* 519–522.

Alcohol-Related Emergencies

8

I. Prevalence and Epidemiology

A. Substance-related emergencies are among the most common psychiatric disorders in the United States. In a recent epidemiological survey (Kessler, et al, 1997), the approximate lifetime rate of alcohol abuse is 9.4% and alcohol dependence was 14.1% of the population. Additionally, the lifetime prevalence of drug abuse is about 4.4% and drug dependence was 7.5% of the population.

B. Alcohol is found relatively constantly throughout the psychiatric emergency services.

C. Substance use disorders are common among clients who present to psychiatric emergency services. Substance use can exacerbate psychiatric symptoms and precipitate a psychiatric emergency. For these reasons, clinicians often face difficult and complex decisions about substance misuse in clients who present with psychiatric symptoms.

D. Research studies confirm that youth of increasingly younger age are using alcohol and illicit substances. Substance-related disorders in this population increases the risk of morbidity and mortality and are often comorbid with other psychiatric disorders.

E. Substance-related disorders mimic numerous psychiatric and medical conditions suggesting the importance of ruling out other psychotic disorders, mania, and anxiety disorders.

F. A large percentage of clients using cocaine are dependent on alcohol (a toxic combination because of neurotoxic and cardiotoxic properties of each drug).

G. Alcohol and other substance use represent a significant risk factor for violence usually during severe intoxication or delirium. Additionally, domestic violence, and an estimated 30% to 50% of child abuse cases involve alcohol and drugs (Collins & Messerschmidt, 1993; Greenfield, 1998; Richardson & Budd, 2003).

H. Alcohol withdrawal delirium is the most serious complication of alcohol withdrawal. Clinical features of alcohol withdrawal can appear within hours of the last consumption, but delirium normally does not emerge until 2 to 3 days after last drink. Mortality rates associated with delirium tremens have fallen to to 0% to 1% with advances in treatment.

Evaluation: Alcohol-Related Emergencies

1. The evaluation of alcohol- and substance-related disorders is an important skill to clinicians because these clients present in the ED with medical, surgical, and psychiatric complications. When a client presents with acute intoxication or other substance-related emergencies, maintaining client and staff safety and medical stability are priorities. Medical complications include overdose, withdrawal or intoxication, withdrawal

seizures, respiratory depression, and cardiac and neurological disturbances. Chronic alcohol use often results in several medical conditions including malnutrition, alcohol hallucinosis and dementia, and Wernicke's encephalopathy. Surgical complications include trauma or injuries from motor vehicle accidents. Psychiatric manifestations include substance-induced psychosis, depression, suicidal or homicidal thoughts. Suicide attempts in these clients are serious issues and must be assessed continuously. Once the acute emergent situation is cleared, clinicians can proceed with an emergency psychiatric assessment to identify medical and comorbid psychiatric disorders that guide treatment recommendations.

2. Making accurate differential diagnoses and initiating appropriate interventions are essential in managing substance-related emergencies. Comorbid medical complications are common and may include malnutrition, dehydration, fluid and electrolyte imbalance, liver disease, gastrointestinal bleeding, systemic infections and myocardial infarction. History of multiple drug use, past withdrawal syndromes or medical and psychiatric complications, such as withdrawal seizures and major depression, must be thoroughly assessed. When a client presents with multiple drug use, clinicians assess the client's "drug of choice." Frequent multiple drug use includes cocaine and alcohol and cocaine and heroin. Clearly, multiple drug use complicates the client's presentation that makes it difficult to differentiate symptoms of intoxication from withdrawal symptoms.

   a. *Differential diagnosis* involves a thorough physical and mental status examination, relevant diagnostic and laboratory studies (i.e., blood alcohol level), Breathalyzer, MSE and CAGE questionnaire. A large number of clients presenting for substance related disorders exhibit some symptoms of depression. These clients must be assessed for comorbid psychiatric and medical conditions, including pregnancy.

Clinicians must ascertain the client's current medical treatment, including all medications—both prescribed and over-the-counter. Clinicians must also inquire about recent accidents, head trauma, fight and major medical and psychiatric conditions. (*See* **CAGE Questionnaire**.)

b. Safe treatment of clients presenting with drug overdoses must take place in a hospital setting, such as the intensive care unit, particularly if the client has severe respiratory depression or coma (APA, 1995).

c. Alcohol is the most common drug used by clients who use emergency services. Causative factors of alcohol related emergencies include both intoxication and withdrawal.

1. *Acute alcohol intoxication* results in impaired cognitive function, poor judgment, disinhibition, increased risk of violence, incoordination, and other altered mental states. Violence often manifests in the form of suicidal or homicidal ideations and behaviors. Alcohol also complicates psychiatric disorders, such as schizophrenia and antisocial personality disorders, by exacerbating the clinical presentation. Intoxicated clients should never be ignored because it is a potentially serious condition and in some cases this can result in coma and death.

CAGE QUESTIONNAIRE

C — Have you felt the need to cut down on your drinking?
A — Have people annoyed you by criticizing your drinking?
G — Have you ever felt bad or guilty about your drinking?
E — Have you had a drink the first thing in the morning to steady your nerves or get rid of a hangover (Eye-opener)?

A score of 2 positive items strongly suggest a need for an in-depth assessment

Physical Examination is likely to reveal a history of recent ingestion of alcohol and the following findings:

- alcohol on breath (mild to moderate intoxication)
- slurred speech
- diminished motor coordination
- ataxia
- unsteady gait
- nystagmus
- impaired attention or memory
- stupor or coma (severe intoxication) (APA, 2000)
- dizziness
- blurred vision
- slurred speech
- flushed face
- hypotension (low blood pressure)
- respiratory depression
- or vomiting
- *Laboratory findings:* elevated blood alcohol level, liver enzymes (AST and ALT), uric acid, serum electrolytes including glucose (to rule out diabetic ketoacidosis) and triglycerides. If there is evidence of blood from stools or vomits—complete blood count (CBC) may reveal anemia
- *Neurological examination,* particularly if client loses consciousness to rule out subdural hematoma and chronic neurotoxic effects, including dementia.

Mental Status Findings—clinical presentations include:

- agitated and uncooperative
- inappropriate (disinhibition) emotional responses
- shortened and impaired attention and memory

- irrational
- angry
- violent
- mood swings
- suicidal ideations*

* Sometimes transitory. When sobriety is reached individual no longer express these thoughts.

Alcohol withdrawal is a serious medical condition that requires early recognition and management. Clients with a history of fatigue, malnutrition, medical conditions, and previous histories of alcohol withdrawal syndromes are predisposed to this serious medical condition. Major stages of alcohol withdrawal are uncomplicated, moderate to severe, severe alcohol withdrawal syndrome and delirium tremens. Characteristic alcohol withdrawal symptoms occur within 4–12 hours after cessation or reduction in alcohol consumption and include:

1. *Uncomplicated alcohol withdrawal* is likely to peak 24 to 48 hours after last drink and subside within 7 days. Major symptoms include mild irritability, tremulousness, anxiety, mild gastrointestinal (GI) disturbances and sleep disturbances that may last about 10 days or longer. Milder forms of uncomplicated withdrawal in the absence of serious medical conditions may subside without treatment. Upon discharge clinicians must make appropriate referrals and dispositions that include health teaching about alcohol and community based mental health services.

2. *Moderate to severe* form: (*See* Physical Examination)

3. *Complicated or severe alcohol withdrawal* often occurs in clients with a 5–15 year history of heavy alcohol use (women about half this time). (See Physical Examination)

4. *Delirium tremens (DTs)* is the major acute complication of alcohol withdrawal, It is a delirium that emerges after cessation of

heavy alcohol use (within 48 hours). Major symptoms include profound autonomic hyperactivity (i.e., increased blood pressure, tachycardia, and diaphoresis). A history of DTs is a predictor of this life threatening medical disorder.

Physical Examination is likely to reveal (moderate to severe withdrawal—onset is usually 24-72 hours of cessation of drinking).

- autonomic hyperactivity (diaphoresis or sweating and pulse > 100 and elevated blood pressure)
- fever
- sleep disturbances
- shakiness and tremulousness (jitteriness)
- nausea or vomiting
- intense anxiety
- grand mal seizures
- poor hydration
- elevated blood pressure
- enlarged or tender liver
- easily bruised
- signs of an infection

Mental Status Examination is likely to reveal (Severe manifestations)

- comatose or stuporous state
- disorientation
- waxing and waning of symptoms
- confusion
- attentional deficits
- perceptual disturbances-especially visual and or tactile hallucinations and delusions
- intense anxiety and agitation

Management of Alcohol-Related Emergencies

I. Psychosocial Interventions—Intoxication

Because clients experiencing alcohol-related emergencies are unpredictable, initiating interventions that maintain staff safety must be a priority. These clients are often cognitively impaired and are at high risk of impulsive and violent behaviors. Loud talking, intrusiveness, pacing, glaring eye contact, and intimidating or threatening remarks signal an emergent situation. The following suggestions will minimize personal violence:

- Assess the client in an open and safe place (avoid isolation that increases the risk of personal violence).
- Assess the client's level of dangerousness to self and other.
- Speak in a calm, yet firm manner.
- Provide generalized support and reassurance.
- Afford close observation and reduce environmental stimuli as needed.
- Provide reorientation and reality testing.
- Assess for signs of withdrawal.
- Approach the client with caution, but be able to muster up help when indicated. Use firm and consistent limit setting and speak in a direct and concise manner.
- Enlist the help of security when the client exhibits verbal escalation to reduce physical threats.
- Use non threatening body language—normal voice tone, eye contact (non glaring) and maintain a safe distance between self and the client.
- Avoid touching or making sudden movements towards the agitated or threatening clients.

- Continuously assess the client's level of dangerousness to self and others because of the high risk of suicide and impulsivity.

Psychosocial Interventions

Withdrawal/DTs (Moderate to severe alcohol withdrawal) include the following:

- A calm and reassuring and nonjudgmental approach
- Afford generalized support and reassurance
- Provide frequent monitoring
- Frequent reorientation
- Around the clock or continuous observation (should never be left alone)
- Assess the client's level of dangerousness to self and others
- Restraints should be used only for short periods—4-point restraints require close observation and relief offered every hour (physical restraint can be minimized by using pharmacological interventions in a timely manner)
- Because of the unpredictable course of these syndromes, their mental and physical status must be constantly assessed. (*See* Chapter 7 for an in-depth discussion)

Pharmacological Interventions

General Considerations

The *goal* of *pharmacological interventions* is to reduce central nervous system (CNS) irritability (seizures), promote sedation, and restore physiological homeostasis. Major strategies include rehydration, benzodiazepines (BDZs), and other medications, such as thiamine and multivitamins. Furthermore, the choice of using pharmacological interventions depends upon the client's presentation-physical and mental status. BDZs remain the treatment of choice for the management of the alcohol withdrawal syndrome. These drugs have a wide margin of safety and are generally well-tolerated.

Benzodiazepines are normally used to treat agitation and anxiety in the intoxicated client. Specific dosing relates to the amount of BDZ necessary to reduce CNS irritability and control vital signs or autonomic hyperactivity in the initial 24 hours.

- After stabilization BDZs are given in four divided doses the following day, and thereafter the dose is tapered over a 5–7 day period.
- Close monitoring during this period for recurrence of symptoms is also part of the treatment protocol.
- Clients with a history of severe alcohol withdrawal and withdrawal-related syndromes may require up to 10 days before BDZs are completely tapered.
- Once detoxification is complete BDZs should be discontinued.

Once *severe alcohol withdrawal* is diagnosed, medical interventions must be initiated to minimize the deleterious progression of this potentially life-threatening syndrome and prevent delirium tremens (DTs). Most facilities have protocols to manage moderate to severe alcohol withdrawal syndromes. These clients may require rehydration, usually intravenous fluids, correction of electrolyte and glucose disturbances, and other symptom management The client's medical status often determines whether long or short-acting benzodiazepines are administered because of compromised liver function. Several strategies are used to determine loading dose, fixed dose, and symptom-triggered methods and include the Clinical Institute Assessment for Alcohol (CIWA-Ar) (Sullivan, et al, 1989).

Common pharmacological protocols include administration of a long-acting BDZ, such as chlordiazepoxide (Librium) every 2 to 4 hours to stabilize the client's medical condition. The usual oral loading dose of chlordiazepoxide is 200–400mg and then 50 mg every 2–4 hours. Short-acting BDZ, such as lorazepam (Ativan), usually 1 mg every 2 hours.

The major advantage of long-acting BDZs is that they allow for "self-tapering" due to cumulative metabolites without a need for more BDZs. Clients experiencing severe withdrawal are given BDZs until withdrawal symptoms and the client's condition stabilize. However, primary disadvantages are these cumulative metabolites that can produce adverse effects in older adults and those with compromised liver/function increase the risk of ataxia, confusion, and oversedation. Another serious disadvantage of long-acting agents is that the IV or intramuscular (IM) route has an unpredictable absorption rate.

In contrast, the short-acting BDZs, such as lorazepam or oxazepam (Serax) are safe and preferred for older clients and those with liver dysfunction, dementia or other cognitive disorders because of fewer cumulative metabolites. Moreover, these agents are readily and reliably absorbed parentally, IV and IM, and rapidly metabolized and eliminated by the kidneys. Frequent dosing and resultant high risk of addiction are the primary disadvantage of the short-acting BDZs.

BDZs are the primary treatment because they decrease the incidence of alcohol withdrawal seizures and DTs. Neuroleptic agents should be avoided because they will lower the seizure threshold and increase the risk of withdrawal seizures. Dosages must be individualized according to the client's presenting symptoms so they can reduce the amount of medication. Most facilities have established protocols for managing alcohol withdrawal syndrome. Management of clients with the alcohol withdrawal syndrome also includes administration of thiamine and magnesium and folate supplementation when indicated.

Disposition

1. *Alcohol Intoxication.* Because alcohol intoxication is time-limited, most clients are discharged to outpatient care. Prior to discharge, assess the client's level of dangerousness and overall psychiatric and medial status. Provide health teaching to the client and family and provide follow up information and referrals for community-based mental health services.

2. *Moderate to Severe Alcohol Withdrawal.* Stuporous or delirious clients are best managed in intensive medical settings because of the risk of seizures, cardiac disturbances, pneumonia and aspiration. Delirium tremens or severe alcohol withdrawal syndrome is also a serious medical manifestation of alcohol withdrawal. Left untreated the severe form of this syndrome can result in death. Additionally, clients who report a history of alcohol withdrawal syndrome require closer observation and prompt medical management of impending symptoms.

3. Hospitalization is also indicated for medical detoxification, especially if there is a history of severe withdrawal syndrome and withdrawal seizures. If there is a negative history of these conditions an outpatient referral detoxification is generally made.

4. Dually-diagnosed clients must be appropriately assessed and evaluated and this data must be used for the basis of community referrals.

5. The *disposition and treatment of children and adolescents* presenting with substance-related emergencies is similar to basic tenets of emergency assessment and treatment of other populations. If the youth poses an acute danger to self and others because of comorbid conditions, inpatient psychiatric hospitalization is indicated. If the child's home setting is unsafe, other measures related to child protective services are needed.

a. Overall, clinicians must assess the level of risk, collaborate with interdisciplinary staff and medical consultants to determine the appropriate disposition.

b. Considerations for disposition and referral must involve the youth's and family's needs and ability to care for the child, and available community referral resources.

Suggested Reading

American Psychiatric Association (2000). *Diagnostic and statistical manual of mental disorders, 4th edition, text revision.* Washington, DC: American Psychiatric Association.

American Psychiatric Association (1995). Practice guideline for the treatment of patients with substance use disorders: Alcohol, cocaine, opioids. *Journal of American Psychiatry, 152,* 5–59

Antai-Otong, D. (1995) Helping the alcoholic patient recover. *American Journal of Nursing, 95* 22–30.

Breslow, RE; Klinger, BI; Erickson, AJ (1996). Acute intoxication and substance abuse among patients presenting to a psychiatric emergency service. *General Hospital Psychiatry, 18,* 183–191.

Collins, JJ & Messerschmidt, PM (1993). Epidemiology of alcohol-related violence. *Alcohol Health Research World, 17,* 93–100.

Dhossche, D; Rubinstein, J (1996). Drug detection in a suburban psychiatric emergency room. *Annals of Clinical Psychiatry, 8,* 59–69.

Ewing, J (1984). Detecting alcoholism: CAGE questionnaire. JAMA, *252,* 1905–1907.

Fleming, M & Manwell, LB (1998). Brief intervention in primary care settings. *Alcohol Research & Health, 23,* 128–137.

Gasfriend, DR; Renner, JA; Hackett, TP (1997). Alcoholic patients-acute and chronic. In NH Cassem; TA Stern; JF Rosenbaum & MS Jellinek (Eds). *Massachusetts General Hospital Handbook of General Psychiatry, 4th edition* (211–230). St. Louis: Mosby.

Greenfield, LA (1998). Alcohol and crime: An analysis of National Data on the prevalence of alcohol involvement in crime. Washington, DC: Bureau of Justice Statistics.

Kessler, RC; Crum, RM; Warner, LA, et al (1997). Lifetime co-occurrence of DSM-III-R alcohol abuse and dependence with other psychiatric disorders in a national comorbidity survey. *Archives of General Psychiatry, 54*, 313–321.

Mayo-Smith, MF (1997). Pharmacological management of alcohol withdrawal: A meta-analysis and evidenced-based practice guideline: American Society of Addiction Medicine Working Group on Pharmacological Management of Alcohol Withdrawal. *Journal of American Medical Association, 278*, 144–151.

Mayo-Smith, MF, Beecher, LH, Fischer, TL, Gorelick, DA, Guillaume, JL, Hill, A, Jara, G, Kasser, C, & Melbourne, J (2004). Management of alcohol delirium: An evidence-based practice guideline. *Archives of Internal Medicine, 164*, 1405–1412.

Richardson, A & Budd, T (2003). Young adults, alcohol, crime and disorder. *Criminal Behavior and Mental Health, 13*, 5–16.

Sadka, S (1995). Psychiatric emergencies in children and adolescents. In M Allen (Ed.). *Growth and Specialization of Emergency Psychiatry* (pp. 65–77). San Francisco: Jossey-Bass Publishers.

Sullivan, IT, Sykora, K, Schneiderman, J, et al (1989). Assessment of alcohol withdrawal: The revised Clinical Institute Withdrawal Assessment for Alcohol scale (CIWA-Ar). *British Journal of Addiction, 84*, 1353–1357.

Other Drug-Related Emergencies

9

A. Cocaine and Amphetamine-Related Emergencies

Evaluation

1. Commonly abused stimulants include cocaine; methamphetamine, also known as "crystal meth" or "ice;" methylphenidate (Ritalin); and methlenedioxyamphetamine, which is often referred to as *Ecstasy* and *Adam*

2. Cocaine psychosis is similar to amphetamine psychosis, but the former is usually shorter in duration

3. Clinicians must make a *differential diagnosis* by ruling out comorbid medical and psychiatric disorders. A serum or urine toxicology screen is the most effective way to differentiate stimulant intoxication.

4. Clients presenting with stimulant intoxication or withdrawal are at high risk for violent and aggressive behaviors towards self and others

5. Typical manifestations of *cocaine and amphetamine and other stimulant intoxication* include physical and mental status examinations:

Physical Examination

- dilated pupils responsive to light
- anorexia
- hyperactivity
- tachycardia (increased heart rate)
- perspiration (diaphoresis)
- hypertension (elevated blood pressure)
- hyperthermia (elevated temperature)
- tremor
- muscle weakness
- pallor
- flushing
- headache
- rhinitis or sinusitis or nasal ulceration (snorting cocaine)
- bronchitis, hoarseness and dark sputum (freebasing cocaine)
- ataxia
- stroke, severe hypertension, hyperpyrexia, and cardiac arrhythmias (these are the most severe adverse effects)

Mental Status Examination

- intense anxiety (panic-like)
- paranoia
- hostility
- rapid speech and thought processes
- hallucinations—visual and tactile ("coke bugs")
- delusions
- confusions
- body-image distortion
- misperception of people's faces
- suicidal ideations
- high risk for violence and assaultive behavior (*See* chapter 6 for a discussion of substance-induced psychosis/delirium)

Cocaine/Amphetamine Withdrawal is not necessarily related to a medical problem or emergency except for the relief of depression and anxiety. Major symptoms of stimulant withdrawal include, dysphoria (depressed mood), agitation, sleep disturbances, and fatigue.

- *Cocaine*—withdrawal symptoms resolve within 7 days
- *Amphetamine*—most signs of intoxication clear up in 2 to 4 days

Management

Once a differential diagnosis is made of stimulant abuse the appropriate intervention may be initiated. *See* Chapter 6 for the treatment of substance-induced psychosis and this chapter for psychosocial interventions.

Disposition

1. Community referrals for the treatment of substance misuse are appropriate.

2. Health teaching about the effects of drugs is an integral part of referral and it must involve family members.

3. Hospitalization is indicated to stabilize the client's medical and psychiatric condition.

B. Opioid-Related Emergencies

Evaluation

1. Commonly abused opioid or narcotics are heroin, oxycontin, meperidine (Demerol), and codeine.

2. Common opioid-related psychiatric emergencies usually occur during *acute intoxication, overdose, or withdrawal conditions*. The severity of symptoms or onset of withdrawal symptoms depend upon drug dose and its half-life. Heroin is considered a short-acting opiate, whereas methadone is considered a long-acting drug. Heroin withdrawal peaks within 36–72 hours and may persist for 1–2 weeks. In comparison, methadone withdrawal peaks at 3–5 days and may last 3–4 weeks. Withdrawal from shorter-acting opiates is shorter, but more intense (Jaffe & Martin, 1990).

3. Differential diagnosis with overdose involves ruling out head trauma and other drugs such as sedatives. Opioid overdose is a medical emergency and requires immediate interventions to stabilize this life threatening situation.

4. Ruling out pregnancy is also necessary to discern treatment goals for clients who are either intoxicated or in withdrawal.

5. Children and Adolescents. There is a paucity of data concerning the treatment of children and adolescents with substance-related disorders. Substances can produce acute behavioral and psychological disturbances and impede developmental tasks. Life-threatening or emergency substance-related disorders must be assessed similarly to adults. Major differences include determining whether one or more drugs exist and if its abuse or dependence. Data from the client, parents, family members, social agencies and other sources are critical in making a differential diagnosis. Questions, such as reasons for referral, parental concerns, knowledge of child's drug use patterns, onset, duration and impact on functioning must be obtained. Comorbid psychiatric conditions, such as conduct disorder and attention-deficit/hyperactivity disorder, are common in children and adolescents with substance-related disorders.

Opioid Overdose

Physical Examination

- decreased respirations or apnea (absence of respirations)
- cyanotic (blue) lips
- hypothermia
- bradycardia
- hypotension
- miosis (pinpoint pupils) [if brain damage has occurred pupils will be dilated] meperidine (Demerol) may also produce dilated pupils
- recent needle marks
- cardiac arrythymias

Mental Status Examination

- comatose
- semicomatose

Management

Pharmacological Interventions

1. The immediate concern in opioid overdose is central nervous depression, which suppresses respiratory centers in the brain stem and medulla

2. Initiate life support appropriate for client's medical condition and presentation (i.e., establish airway, intravenous (IV) access, monitor cardiac status). More importantly, advanced life support should be available along with close monitoring of vital signs)

3. Opioid overdose is a life-threatening situation and warrants immediate treatment with intravenous (IV) naloxone (Narcan), a narcotic receptor antagonist.

    a.   Naloxone (Narcan) 2 mg and then 2–4 mg as needed

    b.   Absence of respiratory depression: 0.4. mg to 0.8 mg and if no response give 2 mg and repeat PRN (as needed) (optimal response occurs within 2–3 minutes after IV injection; 15 minutes after IM, SQ injection

    c.   Recognize that naloxone (Narcan) is more shorter acting than opiates and there is a risk of the client falling back into a coma or becoming apneic (respirations cease)

Disposition

1. Refer for hospitalization and further evaluation and treatment. Close medical observation is critical for at least 24 hours with short-acting opiates and up to 72 hours for long-acting agents.

2. Consider hospitalization for medically unstable clients

3. Refer other clients to traditional treatment programs

Opioid Withdrawal

1. The acute cessation of opiates produces an uncomfortable, but not life-threatening, syndrome unless the client has comorbid medical conditions, such as severe coronary artery disease.

2. Opioid withdrawal is associated with feelings of suspiciousness, hostility and confusion and high risk of violent or aggressive behaviors.

3. Opioid withdrawal symptoms are likely to emerge after abrupt abstinence from *heroin or morphine* after 1 to 2 weeks of continuous use. Withdrawal symptoms appear within 6 to 8 hours, peak on the second or third day, and abate by day 10. Shorter acting narcotics, such as *meperidine* (Demerol) symptoms occur more rapidly and appear within 3 to 4 hours, and peak within 8 to 12 hours, abating within 4 to 5 days.

4. Untreated opioid withdrawal syndrome subsides within 5 to 10 days.

5. Differential diagnosis—rule out alcohol or benzodiazepine withdrawal. Drug screens with urine or serum are helpful in making a differential diagnosis.

Physical Examination

- diaphoresis (sweating)
- rhinorrhea (runny nose)
- tearing
- nausea
- vomiting
- dilated pupils
- sleep disturbances
- decreased appetite
- "goose bumps"
- shakes
- tachycardia
- diarrhea
- aching "all over"
- increased blood pressure
- tachycardia
- abdominal cramps

Mental Status Examination

- anxiety
- craving for opiate (drug seeking—behavior)
- irritability
- agitation
- restlessness
- dysphoria

Management

Clients presenting with opioid withdrawal tend to be very demanding, exhibit drug-seeking behavior and are uncooperative. Clinicians can allay anxiety and agitation by approaching the client cautiously and reassuring him or her that efforts will be used to minimize discomfort, even though they cannot be eliminated. The following interventions are useful in reducing the severity of opioid withdrawal symptoms:

Psychosocial Intervention

1. Approach in a nonjudgmental and supportive manner
2. Assess level of dangerousness to self and others
3. Assess educational needs and provide health teaching

Pharmacological Interventions

1. Catapres (Clonidine), an alpha2 antagonist, is the primary agent used in the treatment of opiate withdrawal. Some clients can be successfully treated with low doses, such 0.1 mg tid. The initial regimen is up to 0.2 mg every 4 hours in clients being managed in outpatient settings Successful outcomes using this approach increase with mild opioid dependence and higher motivation (O'Connor, et al, 1997).

2. A major side effect of catapres (Clonidine) issedation and *hypotension*. (Hypotension [low blood pressure]) needs to be closely monitored.)

3. A contemporary method of opioid withdrawal is a combination of catapres (Clonidine) and naltrexone (ReVia) that produces a more rapid detoxification, despite more intense initial withdrawal than Clonidine alone.

4. Detoxifications usually involves the substitution and tapering of a long-acting opioid, such as methadone. Buprenorphine is a newer and cost-effectve option for detoxification of opioid dependence. This drug produces a low level of physical

dependence and is less likely to cause overdose and produce fewer withdrawal symptoms in comparison to methadone.

Disposition

Refer to a formal drug rehabilitation treatment program and other mental health services when appropriate

C. Benzodizepine-Related Emergencies

Evaluation

1. Benzodiazepines can produce physiological and psychological dependency when used in high doses or in prolonged abuse.

2. Benzodiazepines with a rapid onset of action, such as diazepam (Valium) and alprazolam (Xanax) are drugs of choice for clients with addictive tendencies.

3. Regardless, if the client takes these agents for medically sound reasons under the supervision of a physician, or uses them largely to get high—physiologic or psychologic dependency may occur.

Benzodiazepine (BDZ) Intoxication

1. Clinicians also must assess the reasons for the overdose and rule out suicide attempt particularly when they are taken with other CNS depressants, such as alcohol.

2. Differential diagnosis must include a complete physical and mental status examinations to rule out other psychiatric and medical conditions, including alcohol intoxication. Drug screens and other diagnostic tests must be performed to make

an accurate diagnosis and guide treatment interventions. When excessive amounts are taken by mouth, BDZs rarely cause serious toxicity unless mixed with other CNS depressants, such as alcohol or barbiturates. Usually signs of serious toxicity strongly suggest that another drug was taken as well. Intravenous toxicity is likely to be life-threatening.

Physical and mental status examinations will reveal the following findings:

Physical Examination

- slurred speech
- incoordination
- lethargy
- unsteady gait
- nystagmus
- stupor or coma (APA, 2000)
- hypotension (low blood pressure)
- hypothermia (low temperature)

Mental Status Examination

- Similar to findings in alcohol intoxication

Management
Pharmacological Interventions

BDZ overdose or toxicity is a medical emergency and requires similar interventions to the client who presents with an opioid overdose. Oral BDZs may be removed by ingesting activated charcoal; dialysis may be required when severe symptoms exist. Similarly to opioid overdose, the primary concern about BDZ overdose is its effects on the central nerv-ous system (CNS), specifically depressant properties. Respirations and other physiologic functions must be closely monitored.

The use flumazenil (Romazicon) a BDZ antagonist in the treatment of severe BDZ overdose is controversial. The most serious adverse effects of flumazenil is precipitation of seizures, particularly clients who are dependent on benzodiazepines or those taking tricyclic antidepres-sants (i.e. desipramine).

Psychosocial Interventions

Psychosocial interventions for BDZ are the same as *other CNS depressants*.

Disposition

1. BDZ overdose is a medical emergency and requires intensive care unit admission to further evaluate and treat this life-threatening condition.

Benzodiazepine Withdrawal

1. Two major concerns for clients presenting with BDZ with-drawal are a withdrawal syndrome and serious medical com-plications including seizures

2. Left untreated, this life-threatening condition may result in delirium, withdrawal seizures, and death.

3. The severity of withdrawal syndrome varies according to the dosage of medication used, duration, and last use.

4. The course of withdrawal symptoms is variable. Normally, symptoms occur 2–3 days after last use in short-acting agents, such as alprazolam, but with long-acting agents, symptoms occur 5–6 days after cessation.

5. The differential diagnosis of BDZ withdrawal is similar to other drugs and requires ruling out psychiatric conditions, such as anxiety disorders, alcohol-related withdrawal and other medical causes of delirium. Clinicians should suspect BDZ withdrawal when the client asks for a sedative, exhibits agitation, and has abnormal vital signs. (*See* **Table XII.**) The following presentations are commonly found in BDZ withdrawal:

Physical Examination

- nausea and vomiting
- weakness or lethargy
- delirium
- muscle twitching
- grand mal seizures
- diaphoresis
- hypertension (high blood pressure)
- tachycardia (increase in pulse rate > 100)
- sleep disturbances
- hand tremor (APA, 2000)

Table XII: Benzodiazepines: Duration of Action

Long-Acting Agents: 20 hours or more	Short-Acting Agents: 6 to 19 hours
• Chlordiazepoxide (Librium) (intermediate onset) • Diazepam (Valium) (rapid onset) • clonazepam (Klonopin) (rapid onset)	• lorazepam (Ativan) (intermediate onset) • alprazolam (Xanax) (rapid onset) • oxazepam (Serax) (slow onset)

Mental Status Examination

- anxiety
- agitation
- perceptual disturbances—hallucinations, usually auditory, tactile or visual; illusions

Management

Psychosocial Interventions

1. Reassurance and supportive environment
2. (Same as other substance use disorders)

Pharmacological Interventions

Medical management of BDZ withdrawal symptoms is individualized in accordance with drug type (i.e., drug half life), history of seizures, duration of use and severity of symptoms. During the withdrawal process, client's should be informed of the anticipated temporary worsening of anxiety. Medical management of withdrawal normally includes:

- A gradual dose reduction or tapering over several weeks or months, depending upon the client's symptoms and medication dose or switching to a high-potency, long-acting BDZ, such as clonazepam (Klonopin).
- Most clients tolerate clonazepam very well because of its prolonged self-tapering properties and experience a smoother detoxification course and minimal rebound anxiety.
- Withdrawal from high-potency, short-acting BDZs, such as alprazolam (Xanax) is difficult because rapid tapering, even with a switch to a long-acting high potency agent, allows acute withdrawal symptoms to emerge. Renner & Gastfriend (1997) recommend the following detoxification for BDZ withdrawal schedule:

a. Substitute clonazepam using the ratio of: 0.5 mg of clonazepam for each 1 mg of alprazolam

b. Continue clonazepam for 1–3 weeks (a drug taper is unnecessary because of its self-tapering properties—usually 2–3 weeks.

c. Because of the risk of withdrawal seizures after abrupt discontinuance of clonazepam, clients must be monitored and informed of the possibility

Disposition

1. Once the client is medically stable referral to an intensive outpatient treatment program is indicated to monitor the client's response to tapering

2. Health education for both the client and significant others regarding anticipated anxiety, criteria for seeking medical follow up

3. If other comorbid psychiatric disorders exist, refer for psychiatric management

D. Hallucinogen-Related Emergencies

1. Hallucinogens are commonly used drugs, especially among adolescents and adults.

2. One of the most commonly used hallucinogenic is d-lysergic acid diethylamine (LSD).

Evaluation-Intoxication

1. These drugs produce a dream-like state accompanied by perceptual distortions and vivid hallucinations. Use of these solvents can be dangerous and induce intensely frightening and paranoid states that increase the risk of violent and aggressive behaviors directed towards self and others.

2. Toxic reactions to LSD are generally psychological and produce "bad trips." These symptoms tend to precipitate seeking emergency services.

3. Hallucinogens also complicate psychiatric disorders and clinicians must make differential diagnoses to rule out substance-related, medical and psychiatric disorders.

4. The onset of action of LSD occurs within an hour of ingestion and peaks in 2 to 4 hours, and symptoms endure 8 to 12 hours. Drug screens are helpful in ruling out other drugs, but will not confirm recent use because it only takes a minute amount to produce symptoms of intoxication.

5. The effects of hallucinogens are diverse, variable, and complex and produce profound psychological and physiologic effects ranging from kaleidoscope imaging to activation of the autonomic nervous system (i.e., tachycardia, elevate blood pressure). The recent use of a hallucinogen is likely to produce an array of symptoms.

Physical Examination

- tachycardia
- mydriasis (pupil dilation)
- blurred vision
- tremors
- elevated blood pressure

- incoordination
- diaphoresis (sweating)
- palpitations (APA, 2000)
- death results from cardiac or cerebrovascular disease related to hypertension or hyperthermia or accidental physical injury stemming from poor judgment

Mental Status Examination

- perceptual changes—sense of wakefulness, visual hallucinations
- anxiety
- labile mood and emotional states
- depression
- paranoia
- suspiciousness
- impaired judgement
- ideas of reference
- desperation
- agony
- euphoria
- bliss
- depersonalization, derealization
- agitation
- terrifying feelings and thoughts
- a sense of hopelessness

Management

Psychosocial Interventions

1. Reassure the client that symptoms will clear up in 4 to 8 hours
2. Orient as needed and use "talking down" techniques
3. Speak in a firm, but caring voice
4. Reduce environmental stimuli-keep in quiet room
5. Engage significant others to reassure and comfort the client by talking to him/her in a non threatening manner
6. Encourage to open eyes to reduce "trip"
7. Assess the client's level of dangerousness to self and others and anticipate aggressive behaviors and initiate safety measures
8. Assess health teaching needs when appropriate and educate about the effects of these agents

Pharmacological Interventions

1. Pharmacological interventions are used to treat agitation as needed—usually BDZs
2. BDZs such as lorazepam or diazepam are useful in reducing intense anxiety and agitation

Disposition

1. Once medically and psychiatrically stable, discharge to family and make appropriate community referrals for substance-related rehabilitation
2. If a child or adolescent, refer for family therapy to deal with underlying issues that may contribute to drug use

Hallucinogen Withdrawal

1. Withdrawal from these drugs does not produce serious alterations in the client's physical status. Symptoms tend to be more psychological and include agitation, anxiety and depression.

2. Differential diagnosis is consistent with evaluations of other clients seeking emergency psychiatric treatment. Toxicology screens are useful in ruling out other drug use.

Disposition

1. Once the client is medically and psychiatrically stable, treatment depends upon the presence of comorbid psychiatric or medical conditions and the client's preference

2. Referrals for outpatient substance or psychiatric treatment rehabilitation

E. Other Drug-Related Emergencies

Table XIII: Other Substance-Related Emergencies

Inhalant-Related Emergencies	Anabolic Steroid Abuse
Evaluation	Evaluation
1. Inhalants are usually consumed with a tube, plastic bag, can, or soaked rag through the mouth or nose 2. Nitrous oxide-that has increased up to 50% among youth ages 18–24	1. Clients who use these drugs to enhance their endurance and strength and those who are prone to violence (i.e., athletes, adolescents, young men)

Table XIII: Other Substance-Related Emergencies *(Continued)*

Inhalant-Related Emergencies	Anabolic Steroid Abuse
since 1994. The death rate from this inhalant is increasing. Other examples include gasoline, paint thinner and other aerosols 3. Use of inhalants is usually short-lived 4. These agents are rapidly absorbed through the lungs and delivered to the brain. 5. The effects of inhalants occur within 5 minutes of and may last for 30 minutes to several hours-based on the dose and duration of inhalation. Alcohol tends to enhance the intensity and duration of these agents. For these reasons, these clients are high risk for violence 6. Inhalants are detectable in the blood for 4 to 10 hours after use-toxicology drug screens can confirm the diagnosis. Baseline labs should also be obtained including ECG to rule out medical and psychiatric disorders. Recent inhalation often produces the following presentations:	2. Initial use of anabolic steroids produce euphoria and hyperactivity. Steroids are addictive substances. Examples of these agents include: nandrolone (Durabolin); stanozolol (Winstrol) 3. Researchers submit that there is a link between the use of these drugs and violence. Extensive alcohol use is associated with anabolic steroid use. Clinicians must do a comprehensive medical, drug use history and mental status and make differential diagnosis. Cholesterol screening may reveal increased LDL and decreases HDL (good cholesterol) 4. Heavy use is associated with increased violence
Inhalant Intoxication	**Physical Examination** • acne • abnormal cholesterol levels • abnormal liver function tests • increased muscle mass • edema
Physical Examination • nystagmus • slurred speech • dizziness • cardiac arrythymias* • hepatitis* • renal failure* • lethargy • generalized muscle weakness • blurred vision diplopia • tremor • nausea	**Mental Status Examination** • mania • preoccupation with androgen use • aggressive behavior "roid rage" • depression • anger • somatization • anxiety **Management/Disposition** • Approach in non judgement manner

Table XIII: Other Substance-Related Emergencies (*Continued*)

Inhalant-Related Emergencies	Anabolic Steroid Abuse
• depressed reflexes • delirium • stupor or coma (APA, 2000) • rash and irritation around nose and mouth • unusual breath odor • residue on face, hands, clothes * serious physical consequences **Mental Status Examiniation** • unsteady gait • euphoria • apathy • impaired judgement • impulsive and aggressive behavior • intense anxiety-short lived **Management/Disposition** 1. Management is according to client's presentation and symptoms. If medically or psychiatrically unstable-hospitalization is indicated 2. BDZs are given to relief agitation and intense anxiety 3. When stable-assess health teaching needs and refer for psychiatric treatment if indicated 4. Adolescents require family therapy and appropriate treatment program	• Recognize safety and initiate protective measures • Assess for underlying psychiatric disorder-treat underlying disorder if present • No specific treatment • Health education about long term effects

Suggested Reading

Ahmadi, J (2003). Methadone versus buprenorphine maintenance for the treatment of heroid-dependent outpatients. *Journal of Substance Abuse Treatment, 24,* 217–220.

American Academy of Child and Adolescent Psychiatry (1997). Practice parameters for the assessment and treatment of children and adolescents with substance use disorders. *Journal of the American Academy of Child and Adolescent Psychiatry, 36* (suppl), 140S–156S.

American Psychiatric Association (2000). *Diagnostic and Statistical Manual of Mental Disorders, 4th edition, text revision.* Washington, DC: American Psychiatric Association.

Antai-Otong, D. (1998). Minimizing violence in the chemically dependent client: Treatment considerations. *Journal of Addictions Nursing, 10,* 28–33.

Assadi, SM, Hafezi, M, Mokri, A, Razzaghi, EM, & Ghaeli, P (2004). Opioid detoxification using high doses of buprenorphine in 24 hours: A randomized, double-blind, controlled clinical trial. *Journal of Substance Abuse Treatment, 27,* 75–82.

Gandhi, DH, Jaffe, JH, McNary, S, Kavanagh, GJ, Hayes, M & Currens, M (2003). Short-term outcomes after brief ambulatory opioid detoxification with buprenorphine in young heroid users. *Addiction, 98,* 453–462.

Jaffe, JH (1995). Pharmacological treatment of opioid dependence: Current techniques and new findings. *Psychiatric Annals, 25,* 369–375.

Mattick, R; Kimber, J; Breen, C & Davoli, M (2004). Buprenorphine maintenance versus placebo or methadone maintenance for opioid dependence. *Cochrane Database System Review, 3,* CD002207.

Midgley, SJ; Heather, N & Davies, JB (2001). Levels of aggression among a group of anabolic-androgenic steroid users. *Medical Science Law, 41,* 309–314.

O'Connor, PG, Carroll, KM, Shi, JM, Schottenfeld, RS Kosten, TR & Rounsaville, BJ (1997). Three methods of opioid detoxification in a primary care setting. A randomized trial. *Annals of Internal Medicine, 127,* 526–530.

Renner, JA & Gastfriend, DR (1997). Drug addicted patients. In NH Cassem; TA Stern; JF Rosenbaum & MS Jellinek (Eds.). *Massachusetts General Hospital Handbook of General Hospital Psychiatry, 4th edition.* St. Louis: Mosby.

Sporer, KA; Firestone, J & Isaacs, SM (1996). Out-of-hospital treatment of opioid overdose in an urban setting. *Academy of Emergency Medicine, 3,* 660–667.

Mood-Related Emergencies 10

Prevalence and Epidemiology

1. Mood disorders are common.

2. Survey data confirms that the lifetime and 12 months prevalence of affective (mood) disorders in the general population is about 19.3% and 11.3% respectively (Kessler, et al, 1994).

3. The morbidity and mortality of depression are high. Approximately 15% of clients with recurrent depression eventually commit suicide. Because suicidal ideations occurs in about 50% of clients seeking psychiatric emergency care, early diagnosis and treatment the ED has the potential to decrease morbidity (Allen, 1996; Grady, Sederer, & Rothchild, 1997).

4. Bipolar disorders account for a prevalence of only 0.3% to 17% in a national epidemiological survey, yet it accounted for 13.2% of presentations to 51 psychiatric emergency services (Weissman, et al, 1996).

5. The goals of psychiatric emergency care of people with mood disorders are changing. Historically, the care of these clients

was to "evaluate and refer." This standard of emergency care no longer meets the needs of clients, clinicians or communities. Initiating a definitive plan of treatment in the emergency settings is emerging as the standard of care (Allen, 1996).

6. Because of the high prevalence of mood disorders, clinicians must be able to use a comprehensive assessment process and provide initial interventions for clients who present with depression and bipolar disorders.

7. Mood disorders represent the most common psychiatric conditions assessed in the ED. Given that these clients are a high risk for suicide and self-neglect, accurate diagnosis and decision-making are crucial to emergency management.

Evaluation—Depression

1. Clients presenting with major depressive episodes must be assessed for the onset, severity, and duration of symptoms. Clinicians must also assess the overall impact of symptoms on the clients' level of functioning and include evaluating physical, emotional, cognitive, and mood disturbances. Older adults are more likely to complain of somatic complaints rather than a depressed mood. Children and adolescents may present with an irritable rather than sad or depressed mood. Initially asking the client about reasons for seeking emergency services at this time; identifying recent stressors, losses, or lifestyle changes, and assessing present and past coping skills and present level of functioning. Other questions that may elicit this information include:

   • How long have you felt sad, depressed, or anxious?
   • What has worked for you in the past?

- Over the past 6–12 months have you had any changes in your mood, sleeping patterns, energy level, or appetite?

- Is there a family history of depression or other psychiatric disorders? If so, what type of treatment was rendered? Was it helpful?

- Is there a history of a manic episode? Was it treated? If so, how?

2. Because of the high risk of suicide in the client experiencing a major depressive episode, in both unipolar and bipolar disorders, a thorough *suicide and homicide assessment* is imperative. This information must be documented and be the basis for interventions and referral and disposition.

3. *Differential diagnosis* must include information about present physical status, medical and psychiatric histories, including substance-related and anxiety disorders. A comprehensive medical evaluation that includes appropriate diagnostic and laboratory tests. Major medical disorders that produce depressive symptoms include endocrine disorders, such as hypothyroidism, pancreatic cancer, medications—both prescribed and over-the-counter drugs, such as those used to treat high blood pressure (i.e., beta blockers) and reduce gastric acid (i.e., ranitidine [Zantac]). Other comorbid psychiatric disorders must also be ruled out, such as anxiety disorders, bereavement and substance-related disorders—both withdrawal syndromes and intoxication. (See **Table XIV**.)

4. Early and accurate evaluation and treatment of major depressive episodes may reduce morbidity and mortality.

5. *Major symptoms of major depressive episodes* include a mood disturbance—sad or depressed—that meets the DSM-IV, Text Revision (TR) criteria (APA, 2000). Symptoms must be present during the same *2-week period* and reflect a *change in the client's previous level of functioning* and meet at least one of the

Table XIV: Common Medical Conditions Associated With Depressive Symptoms

Medical Conditions	Medications
Endocrine • diabetes mellitus • hypothyroidism • premenstrual dysphoric disorder • postpartum depression • menopause • Addison's disease • Cushing's syndrome	**Cardiac and Antihypertensive agents** • clonidine • digitalis (Lanoxin) • propranolol (Inderal) • prazosin (Minipress) • ace-inhibitors
Neurologic • Alzheimer's disease and other primary dementias • stroke • brain tumors • epilepsy • vascular dementia • Parkinson's disease • Huntington disease	**Steroids and Hormones** • corticosteroids **NSAIDs (non steroidal anti-inflammatory drugs)** • ibuprofen (Motrin) • ranitidine (Zantac)
Metabolic • Vitamin deficiences—B_{12}, folate, niacin, thiamin • electrolyte imbalance-hypokalemia	**Antibacterial Agents** • tetracycline • sulfonamides • streptomycin • ampicillin
Infection/Inflammatory • hepatitis • mononucleosis • tuberculosis • HIV disease • systemic lupus erythematosous (SLE) • Crohn's disease	**Other** • diphenhydramine hydrochloride (Benadryl)
Other • pancreatic and lung cancer • anemias • post MI (heart attack), post heart surgery • renal disease • cancer	

following presentations (*See* Physical and Mental Status Examination findings). Children and adolescents are more likely to present with an irritable mood. The client's symptoms must also produce significant distress that has a global impact and does not meet criteria for other psychiatric or medical conditions.

Physical Examination

- appetite and weight disturbances
- sleep disturbances—insomnia or hypersomnia nearly every day
- fatigue or loss of energy nearly everyday
- decreased libido

Mental Status Examination

- marked diminished interest or pleasure in activities that were once pleasurable
- psychomotor agitation or retardation
- feelings of worthlessness or inadequacy or extreme guilt
- recurrent thoughts of suicide or death
- decreased ability to think or concentrate, or indecisiveness
- social isolation

Management

Once the diagnosis of major depressive episode has been determined appropriate psychosocial and pharmacological interventions should be utilized.

Psychosocial Interventions

1. Use an unhurried approach to establish rapport and assess the meaning of present stressors
2. Afford a supportive approach to convey warmth, empathy and hope
3. Focus on the client's strengths and available support systems and resources
4. Provide health education regarding medications, depressive illness (a treatable disease), and treatment approaches
5. Focus on client's feelings and encourage ventilation
6. Determine the impact of the client's symptoms on his/her level of functioning and potential for danger towards self and others

Pharmacological Interventions

1. Once a diagnosis of depression is determined and after health education about the disorder has been made—pharmacological agents can be prescribed. Glick (2000) suggest that clinicians prescribing these agents should also use the following general principles:

   • Provide only enough medication for several days at a time, with follow-up arrangement accordingly

- A follow-up plan is necessary prior to starting the antidepressant
- When a short follow-up appointment is unavailable the client should return to the ED for re-evaluation within 2–3 days
- Clear documentation of reasons for prescribing antidepressants is imperative along with reasons for a specific agent, health teaching, and follow-up plan
- Communicate with follow-up clinician that will be treating client with the client's written permission only. If the client is unwilling to give permission, medications should not be initiated in the ED
- Assess health teaching needs—educate about depression, medication/other treatment—including reason, duration, and side effects.

2. With the advent of newer antidepressant agents, clinicians now have a broader range of medications, many of which have a safer side effect and overdose risk profile. Despite their efficacy, tricyclic antidepressants are likely to produce serious and potentially fatal side effects including cardiotoxicity and high risk for lethal overdoses. Newer agents include selective serotonin reuptake inhibitors (SSRIs), such as fluoxetine (Prozac) and the serotonin norepinephrine reuptake inhibitors, such as venlafaxine (Effexor) are safer in overdose, generally well tolerated, and less prone to produce cardiovascular side effects (Ellison & Pfaelzer, 1995). Clinicians prescribing antidepressants should consider:

- client preferences
- history of response (client or biologic relative)
- safety (lethality in overdose)
- side effects (long-term safety and tolerability)

- interactions with comorbid conditions and drugs
- cost (affordability)
- neurotransmitter specificity

3. *Children and adolescents.* The decision to initiate antidepressant treatment versus specific psychotherapy is made collaboratively with the clinician and informed parents or guardians with agreement from the youth. The first line treatment for youth are the SSRIs that seem to be safe and effective in treating this population (Emslie, et al, 1999). Several researchers (Emslie, et al, 2000; Leonard, et al, 1997) submit that the criteria for determining pharmacological interventions includes several factors:

- Severity of the depression
- Biological family members response to medications
- Recurrence and chronic course of illness
- Poor response to psychotherapy
- Family preference and convenience
- Nature of psychosocial stressors

Disposition

1. Hospitalization is indicated when the client is medically or psychiatrically unstable, including high risk for suicide and psychotic symptoms
2. Outpatient and community referrals for medication management, psychotherapy, crisis intervention, day hospital or other treatment programs.

3. Referral to mobile crisis teams and residential crisis unit is an alternative to hospitalization when the client requires access to immediate support and observation of treatment responses.

4. Referrals for youth may involve pharmacological management and a combination of psychotherapy—family and individual

5. Provide interim support until client able to get community appointment for various treatment referrals

Bipolar Disorder I—Manic Episode

The diagnosis of mania is challenging to most clinicians, particularly when the client presents with a behavioral emergency. The pervasive illicit substance use among these clients complicates the diagnosis and contributes to an increased risk of agitation and aggression.

Evaluation

1. Prompt recognition of bipolar disorder and rapid initiation of appropriate treatment are essential to the appropriate management of mania in psychiatric emergency settings.

2. Normally, concerned family members, law officers, or other mental health providers bring these clients into the ED. Because of the client's lack of insight into his or her illness and the need for treatment, clinicians are challenged to treat behavioral and psychotic symptoms making a differential diagnosis very difficult.

3. Making a *differential diagnosis* involves evaluating and ruling out a general medical condition, drug toxicity or adverse reactions, other psychiatric, such as schizoaffective disorder, and

substance-related disorders in efforts to make a differential diagnosis and initiate appropriate treatment and disposition.

4. Clinicians should also perform a *psychosocial assessment* and gather information about onset and duration of symptoms (i.e., rapid cycling, depressed states, mixed), past and present treatment, present and past coping patterns, including suicide or homicide risk, and substance misuse history and treatment. The clients are commonly unreliable historians, and efforts to obtain information from other sources are imperative. It should also include information about side effects or adverse drug reactions to previous interventions. Because of the high *risk of violence*, clinicians must initiate protective measures to reduce agitation and protect the client and staff.

5. Given that the client is diagnosed with bipolar disorder, Type I, acute manic episode. The client presents with a distinct period of elated, expansive or irritable mood that lasts for at least one week (APA, 2000) and the following presentation:

Physical Examination

- sleep disturbances-decreased need for sleep
- hypersexuality
- increased energy
- possible weight loss related to client not taking the time to eat

Mental Status Examination

- elated, irritable or expansive mood
- intrusiveness

- pressured speech
- tangentiality or circumstantiality
- flight of ideas
- inflated self-esteem—(delusions of grandeur)
- easily distracted and decreased concentration
- delusions*
- hallucinations*
- impaired judgement
- unreliable historians
- emotional lability
- loose associations

* with psychotic symptoms

Management

The management of bipolar disorder, Type I, manic episode, must focus on alleviating acute symptoms and symptom management. The treatment often requires seclusion, restraint, or hospitalization, but may also be managed on an ambulatory or residential settings depending on the client's clinical presentation. Hospitalization is usually necessary if the client has severe and/or psychotic symptoms or high risk of danger to self or others, or exhibits cognitive disturbances. Less severe symptoms may be manageable in residential settings. First episodes are most likely to require hospitalization to further assess the client's symptoms and facilitate behavioral management.

Psychosocial Interventions

1. Approach the client in a calm, yet firm manner.

2. Use clear, concrete and simple statements.

3. Be cognizant of personal safety and the client's intrusive behavior. Put personal safety before privacy.

4. When offering medications approach with a suggestion rather than order, "Mary, this medication will make it easier for you to regain control over yourself."

5. Continuously assess the client's level of danger to self and others.

6. Reduce environmental stimuli.

7. Use verbal de-escalating techniques and consistent and firm limit setting

8. Consider the use of restraints before behavior escalates as the last resort.

Pharmacological Interventions

1. Clients with acute mania are vulnerable to hyperarousal and they fear loss of control. Pharmacological interventions aid in creating an internal barrier against hyperarousal. Because a 1 to 2 week course is needed for titration and improvement with antimanic agents, managing acute mania requires an approach that facilitates rapid control of behavioral symptoms that includes

   a.   Intramuscular (IM) or oral neuroleptic (i.e., haloperidol) and/or benzodiazepine (BDZ), such as lorazepam, when the client is cooperative, with an oral mood stabilizer, such as valproate acid. BDZs may be useful in managing mild manic episodes, but in severe episodes they may cause behavioral disinhibition (Dubovsky & Buzan,

1997). Antipsychotic and BDZ combination usually improve the client's mood, psychosis, and behavior within several days (Yatham, 2003). Newer atypical antipsychotic agents produce fewer EPS symptoms than typical agents. Some troublesome side effects of these newer agents involve significant weight gain, alterations in lipid levels and abnormalities in glucose tolerance. Moreover, they produce rapid sedation, usually within one to three doses and reduce arousal regardless of the underlying psychiatric disorders. (*See* Chapter 6 for further discussion of pharmacological management of psychotic disorders).

b.   During early treatment with these agents, antimanic agents and.or mood stabilizers are titrated to therapeutic doses. There is growing evidence of the efficacy of anticonvulsant agents in the management of acute mania. Valproate loading of 30 mg/kg/d orally in divided doses for the initial 2 days appears to be one of the safest and most expedient modes to initiation of definitive treatment (Allen, 2000). Prior to beginning this agent, baseline blood counts, liver function tests, and in childbearing women, pregnancy tests are imperative.

Disposition

1. As previously discussed hospitalization is generally the disposition of choice for the client presenting with acute mania. Barriera (1994) delineates criteria for hospitalization when the manic client:

- poses a danger to self and others
- has impaired self care deficits

- is at physical risk of not eating or sleeping
- exhibits psychotic symptoms
- is uncooperative or unwilling to comply with outpatient treatment
- lacks quality support systems
- has a history of poor medication compliance

2. Other referrals may include referral to residential settings, extended care settings if the client is older and resides in this facility.

3. Children and adolescents are likely to require hospitalization for close medication titration and observation for desired and adverse drug reactions and monitoring of sucidality. Family therapy and psychoeducation are integral aspects of the youth's treatment planning.

Suggested Reading

Allen, MH (1996). Definitive treatments in the psychiatric emergency service. *Psychiatric Quarterly, 67,* 247–262.

Allen, MH & Currier, GW (2000). Diagnosis and treatment of mania in the psychiatric emergency service. *Psychiatric Annals, 30,* 258–266.

American Psychiatric Association (2000). *Diagnostic and Statistical Manual of Mental Disorders, 4th edition, Text revision.* Washington, DC: American Psychiatric Association.

Antai-Otong. D. (2001). Dark days: Treating major depression. *Advance for Nurse Practitioners, 9,* 32–33, 37–38, 43.

Belmaker, RH (2004). Bipolar disorder. *New England Journal of Medicine, 351,* 476–486.

Dubovsky, SL & Buzan, RD (1997). Novel alternatives and supplements to lithium and anticonvulsants for bipolar affective disorder. *Journal of Clinical Psychiatry, 58,* 224–242.

Eastham, JH; Jeste, DV & Young, RC (1998). Assessment and treatment of bipolar disorder in the elderly. *Drugs & Aging, 12,* 205–224.

Ellison, JM & Pfaelzer, C (1995). Emergency pharmacotherapy: The evolving role of medications in the emergency department. *New Directions for Mental Health Services, 67,* 87–98.

Emslie, GJ; Walkup, JT; Pliska, SR; et al (1999). Current trends in children and adolescents. *Journal American Academy of Child and Adolescent Psychiatry, 38,* 517–528.

Emslie, GJ; Mayes, TL & Hughes, CW (2000). Updates in the pharmacological treatment of childhood depression. *Psychiatric Clinics of North America, 23,* 813–835.

Glick, RL (2000). Initiation of antidepressant medications in the emergency setting. *Psychiatric Annals, 30,* 251–257.

Grady, TA; Sederer, LI & Rothchild, AJ (1997). Depression. In LI Sederer & AJ Rothchild (Eds). *Acute Care Psychiatry* (pp. 83–121). Baltimore, MD Williams & Wilkins.

Kessler, RC; Nelson, CB; Zhao, S; et al (1994). Lifetime and 12-month prevalence of DSM-III-R psychiatric disorders in the United States: Results from the National Comorbidity Survey. *Archives of General Psychiatry, 51,* 8–19.

Leonard, HL; March, J; Rickler, KC, et al (1997). Pharmacology of the selective serotonin reuptake inhibitors in children and adolescents. *Journal American Academy of Child and Adolescent Psychiatry, 36,* 725–736.

Weissman, MM; Bland, RC; Canino, GJ; et al, (1997). Cross-national epidemiology of major depression and bipolar disorder. *JAMA, 276,* 293–299.

Yatham, LN (2003). Acute and maintenance treatment of bipolar mania: The role of atypical antipsychotics. *Bipolar disorder, 5 Suppl,* 7–19.

Anxiety-Related Emergencies

Epidemiology and Prevalence

1. Anxiety disorders are the most common psychiatric disorders.
2. The lifetime prevalence of any anxiety disorder is 24.9% and the 12-month prevalence is 17.2% (Kessler, et.al., 1994).
3. There is a high prevalence of comorbid anxiety and mood disorders.

Evaluation

1. Assessing the anxious client follows the principles of the psychosocial assessment of all psychiatric clients.
2. *Differential diagnosis* also follows these principles and involves ruling out underlying medical conditions. This process includes ordering appropriate laboratory and diagnostic studies, including an ECG. An array of medical conditions can produce anxiety symptoms. These conditions include endocrine and neurological conditions, systemic conditions,

and myocardial infarction (MI). Other conditions that cause anxiety symptoms include drug toxicity, other psychiatric or substance-related disorders, such as withdrawal or intoxication states and dietary supplements, such as caffeine or dieting agents. Clinicians should *suspect an underlying general medical condition* if symptoms have an acute onset, initial manifestation emerge after age 40, are accompanied by fluctuation in sensorium and hallucinations, and unstable vital signs (Milner, Florence, & Glick, 1999).

3. Assessment of the client's symptoms must include onset, duration, and their impact on the client's level of functioning. Clinicians should elicit information about the course of symptoms—remitting or unremitting, precipitating events, such as those associated with phobias and recurrence. Discerning the client's reasons for seeking treatment and recent stressors and coping skills, also provides understanding about causative factors and potential treatment considerations.

4. Suicide risk must be assessed, particularly if the client reports impaired functional status due to severity and nature of symptoms.

5. Issues such as recent and past traumatic encounters, fears, and avoidant behaviors provide crucial information about specific primary anxiety disorders.

6. Causative and clinical symptoms of anxiety disorders vary, but clients often present characteristic biological, emotional, cognitive and behavioral manifestations. Prominent anxiety, panic attacks, phobias, or obsessions or compulsions are common clinical features of anxiety disorders. The physical and mental status examination of an anxious client often includes:

Physical Examination

- dizziness and lightheadedness
- palpitations
- shaking
- chest pain or discomfort
- abdominal distress
- hypertension
- shortness of breath
- diaphoresis (sweating)
- tachycardia
- increased respirations
- paresthesias (tingling sensations in extremities)
- upset stomach
- muscle tension
- restlessness

Mental Status Examination

- derealization
- depersonalization
- concentration disturbances
- fears (intense)
- avoidant behaviors

(*See* **Table XV.**)

Table XV: Specific Anxiety Disorders and Pharmacological Interventions

Specific Anxiety Disorder	Signs and Symptoms	Pharmacological Interventions
1. Panic disorder— frequent comorbidity of depression and other anxiety disorders	**discrete episode, abrupt onset:** • shortness of breath • dizziness • paresthesias (numbness/tingling) • trembling, shakiness • palpitations • diaphoresis (sweating) • avoidant behaviors • chest pain/discomfort • derealization • fear of losing control, "going crazy" • disorder interferes with global level of functioning	**SSRIs—first line treatment* for panic disorder (PD) due to their relatively favorable side effect profile** • fluoxetine (Prozac) • sertraline (Zoloft) • paroxfetine (Paxil) • citalopram (Celexa) • escitalopram (Lexapro) **BDZs**** (clonazepam [Klonopin]) provides rapid relief and less rebound and withdrawal symptoms than alprazolam (Xanax)
2. Obsessive-compulsive disorder (OCD)	• persistent, intrusive thoughts and images (obsessions) and the client feels driven to perform ritualistic and repetitive behaviors (compulsions) • client realizes the irrational or excessive nature of obsessions and compulsions, but cannot control them. • chronic in nature with few remissions • interfere with global level of functioning	• Clomipramine (a tricyclic antidepressant [TCA] with potent serotonin reuptake inhibitor properties) • SSRIs

Table XV: Specific Anxiety Disorders and Pharmacological Interventions *(Continued)*

Specific Anxiety Disorder	Signs and Symptoms	Pharmacological Interventions
3. Post-traumatic stress disorder (PTSD)	a syndrome that is characterized by responses to an overwhelming traumatic or stressor-(combat battle, rape, assault, life-threatening accidents) • intrusive behaviors-recollections and dreams, flashbacks and nightmares • intense physiological distress • avoidant behaviors • numbness of responsiveness • hyperarousal-sleep disturbances, hypervigilance, startle response	• SSRIs (sertraline [Zoloft]) • topiramate (Topamax)
Generalized anxiety disorder (GAD)	• persistent, chronic, excessive worrying • irritability • sleep disturbances • muscle tension • excessive symptoms impair global functioning	• SSRIs • venlafaxine (Effexor)

(APA, 1994)

Data from Zohar, J & Westenberg, HGM (2000). Anxiety disorders: A review of tricyclic antidepressants and selective serotonin reuptake inhibitors. *Acta Psychiatrica Scandinavica, 101 (Suppl 403)*, 39–49.

* Simon & Pollack (2000)

** BDZs (benzodiazepines)

Management

The principal goal of intervention during psychiatric emergent situations is to reduce the client's anxiety level. This involves psychosocial and pharmacological interventions. The latter depends upon the specific anxiety disorder and comorbid psychiatric and substance-related disorders.

Psychosocial Interventions

1. Approach the client in a calm and unhurried manner
2. Reassure the client that he or she is not "going crazy" or dying by reviewing the result of ECG
3. Encourage to take slow deep breaths and focus on present concerns
4. Provide health education about specific anxiety disorder including precipitants and non-pharmacological interventions

Pharmacological Interventions

1. Specific pharmacological interventions depend upon client's present distress and specific anxiety disorder
2. Benzodiazepines are standard drug treatment for acute symptoms of anxiety disorders and produce their effects within 30 to 60 minutes. High-potency BDZ, such as alprazolam and clonazepam have proven efficacy for panic disorder-they have a rapid onset
3. Currently, the treatment of choice for clients with obsessive compulsive disorder (OCD) is clomipramine and SSRIs, such as fluvoxamine (Luvox)
4. The *first line treatment* of panic disorder in clients with a history of substance abuse who have not been on pharmacother-

apy for their disorder is a combination of a selective serotonin reuptake inhibitor (SSRI), such as paroxetine (Paxil) plus psychotherapy (Brawman-Mintzer & Lydiard, 1996)

5. Clients experiencing generalized anxiety disorder (GAD and/or comorbid major depressive episode) have been successfully treated with venlafaxine (Effexor) XR and SSRIs, such as escitalopram (Lexapro).

(*See* **Table XV.**)

Disposition

1. Hospitalization is limited to clients who are medically unstable and at high risk for danger to self and others

2. Refer client for psychotherapy that focuses on cognitive behavioral therapy, desensitization and pharmacological interventions as appropriate or with comorbid psychiatric disorders, such as major depressive episode

3. Children who present with separation anxiety or other childhood disorders may benefit from family therapy and pharmacological interventions with comorbid psychiatric disorders

4. Clients presenting with post traumatic stress or acute stress disorders will benefit from a referral to local vet centers, rape crisis counselors and support groups, or treatment that provides interventions for trauma survivors

Suggested Reading

American Psychiatric Association (2000). *Diagnostic and Statistical Manual of Mental Disorders, 4th edition, text revision*. Washington, DC: American Psychiatric Association.

Antai-Otong, D (2000). The neurobiology of anxiety disorders: Implications for psychiatric nursing practice. *Issues in Mental Health Nursing, 21*, 71–89.

Brawman-Mintzer, O & Lydiard, RB (1996). Psychopharmacology of anxiety disorders: Treatment resistance. *Psychiatric Clinics of North America, 3*, 66–67.

Goodman, WK; Ward, HE & Murphy, TK (1998). Biological approaches to treatment-refractory obsessive-compulsive disorder. *Psychiatric Annals, 28*, 641–649.

Hackett, D (2000). Venlafaxine XR in the treatment of anxiety. *Acta Psychiatrica Scandinavica, Supplementum, 406*, 30–35.

Kessler, RC; Nelson, CB; Zhao, S; et al (1994). Lifetime and 12-month prevalence of DSM-III-R psychiatric disorders in the United States: Results from the National Comorbidity Survey. *Archives of General Psychiatry, 51*, 8–19.

Matthew, SJ; Simpson, HB; Fallon, BA (2000). Treatment strategies for obsessive-compulsive disorder. *Psychiatric Annals, 30*, 699–708.

Milner, KK; Florence, T & Glick, RL (1999). Mood and anxiety syndromes in emergency psychiatry. *Psychiatric Clinics of North America, 22*, 755–777.

Managing Violence in Psychiatric Emergency Settings

12

Epidemiology and Prevalence

1. Perhaps the single issue that concerns most clinicians is the client at risk for harming others. Violent or aggressive behavior is a common reason that clients are brought to psychiatric emergency settings for evaluation and possible hospitalization.

2. The psychiatric emergency room or triage has become the chief access to acute psychiatric services for clients with severe mental disorders, especially those who are violent.

3. There is a preponderance of research that shows a relationship between mental illness and violence. Data confirms that violent behavior is five times more common in clients with serious mental illnesses, including schizophrenia and mood

disorder, than in controls and 10 to 15 times more prevalent when they have comorbid substance-related disorders (Asnis, Kaplan, Hundorfean, Saeed, 1997; Steadman, Mulvey, Monahan, et al., 1998).

4. A history of violent or criminal behavior is the *best predictor* of violence (*See* **Table XVI.**)

Evaluation

1. Gather as much information about the client as possible to identify violence risk factors through clinical interview

2. Initially, clinicians must recognize that violence can occur any-where, remain calm and non-threatening. Act assertively and decisively and with sufficient and appropriately trained backup when violence is imminent.

Table XVI: High Risk Populations for Violence

- History of child abuse or witnessed domestic violence
- Low intelligence-mentally challenged
- Neurologic impairment-brain injury, seizure disorder
- Dementia and other cognitive disorders
- Psychotic disorders, particularly in the presence of command hallucinations
- Male gender
- Adolescents and early twenties (persons with and without mental illness)
- Personality disorders (i.e., antisocial personality, borderline personality disorder)
- Weapon availability and preoccupation with violent thoughts
- Substance-related disorders-both intoxication and withdrawal states
- Autism-irritability and aggressive behavior
- Children and adolescents with aggressive conduct disorder or attention deficit disorder

3. Ensure staff safety by making sure that the clinician is between the client and the door and that staff is easily accessed during the interview. The psychiatric emergency settings should be free of objects that can be used as a weapon. Have restraints available for acutely agitated clients prior to the formal interview and use as a last resort.

4. Clinicians must attempt to make *differential diagnosis*, particularly when the client is acutely agitated. The clients must be evaluated for delirium and other general medical conditions. Clinicians should order appropriate diagnostic and laboratory studies to rule out medical, psychiatric and substance-related disorders. Suggested laboratory studies include chemistry profile, blood indices, tests for syphilis, toxicology screens, thyroid panel, urinalysis, and liver function tests.

5. Search for weapons. Assess the client for a weapon often involves asking about weapons and using metal detectors. If metal detectors are used an armed guard or police officer should be available otherwise the risk of violence increases if an alarm goes off and no can retrieve it from the client.

   Avoid taking a weapon from the client. Security must be involved in this process to reduce harm to clinician and client.

6. Institute risk assessment principles, such as obtaining a history of violence—including domestic violence, arrests, juvenile court involvement, hospitalization for violent behavior, and substance misuse. A previous history of clinician assault, denial of admission sought by client and recent threats of assault are also clinical indicators of high-risk behaviors. Staff training is necessary to learn methods of assessing, preventing and physical management of dangerous and aggressive behaviors.

7. High-risk clients are likely to be restless and agitated and have fixed facial expression. They are also likely to be verbally profane or threatening. These behaviors should never be ignored. Verbal threats and signs of restlessness and pacing usually pre-

cede physical aggression. Perform a mental status examination immediately and observe the client's posture, mannerisms, appearance, voice tone and rate, orientation, and mode of arrival. Clinicians also need to pay attention to their "gut" reaction and respond accordingly.

Physical Examination

It is difficult to perform a physical examination on a client during the midst of a violent episode. However, efforts to conduct an examination should be done as soon as possible to make a differential diagnosis and initiate appropriate treatment. The results of the physical examination depend upon the underlying cause. The agitated or irritable client is likely to exhibit the following physical manifestations:

- restlessness
- shortness of breath
- tachycardia (increased pulse rate)
- elevated blood pressure
- dilated pupils
- nystagmus
- elevated temperature
- slurred speech
- clenched jaw or fist
- muscle tension
- increased respirations
- diaphoresis
- pacing
- flared nostrils

- flushed face
- hands clenched
- skin lacerations

Mental Status Examination

- psychomotor agitation
- hallucinations
- delusions
- anger
- hostility
- uncooperativeness
- impulsivity
- shouting and cursing
- slamming objects
- suspiciousness
- disorganized thoughts
- impaired judgment and cognition

Management

Psychosocial Interventions

1. Approach the client in a calm and empathetic manner using a normal voice tone. Clinicians can convey respect and concern by introducing oneself and calling the client by name.
2. Discern personal reactions to the client and maintain a non-judgmental approach. Many clinicians feel vulnerable and

143

respond to violent situations with fear, anxiety and frustration. Acutely agitated and psychotic clients are very sensitive to environmental stimuli and are likely to sense the clinician's reactions. In these cases, it is imperative to regain control over one's reactions and seek immediate assistance, because the client is likely to escalate and become physically violent. Clients look to clinicians to help them regain control and a fearful or anxious clinician is likely to aggravate the client's fears and anxiety and risk of violence.

3. Prior to approaching an agitated or restless client, make sure that you are between the client and an exit, mobilize adequate staff support and anticipate physical aggression

4. Consider restraints or seclusion as a last resort

5. Initiate *verbal de-escalation and limit setting* techniques by using a firm and supportive voice tone and providing eye contact. (*See* **Table XVII.**)

- Clinicians should approach the client cautiously and use simple and concise statements and redirect the client who is shouting or yelling and verbalize that they want to help, but violence is unacceptable and describe consequences if it continues or occurs

- Encourage expression of feelings and reasons for being upset.

- Listen to angry clients

- It is imperative for clinicians to recognize their limitations and acknowledge their fears of threatening clients—this can be life saving

- Reorient confused or disoriented clients (never leave them alone)

Table XVII: Behavioral Interventions

Verbal De-escalation:
- Establish empathy
- Use non-threatening body language
- Establish rapport
- Address the client's affect
- Set firm and consistent limits
- Inform "you have a choice. . . . or if you feel out of control you can sit in the seclusion room"

Talk Down Procedures:
- Assess the imminence of escalation
- Determine a plan of escape
- Secure help
- Establish verbal contact
- Make sure the client can hear and respond to you
- Use assertive communication and short sentences

Dealing with Angry Clients:
- Stand on non-dominant side
- Use non-threatening body language
- Avoid glaring eye contact
- Give information in terms of suggestions, rather than demands
- Ensure that a mechanism to muster up help is available
- Secure dangerous objects

- Clinicians should point out that they are there to also help the client regain control

6. When appropriate offer medications—either oral or injection

7. Assess the clients response to interventions

Pharmacological Interventions

1. Pharmacological interventions are required when the client does not respond to psychosocial interventions and verbal de-escalation and limit setting.

2. Initial considerations for pharmacological interventions include the type of agent and route of administration.

3. Normally a neuroleptic (i.e., haloperidol, up to 10 mg) and ben-zodiazepine, such as lorazepam (Ativan) are drugs of choice for managing acute agitation and aggressive behaviors. Lorazepam (2mg) is an ideal drug for acute agitation, particularly when the underlying cause is unknown. This drug can be administered intramuscularly (IM) and is readily absorbed. Specific medica-tion dosing must be in accordance with the client's presenting symptoms, including age, weight and causative factors. It is important when appropriate to ask the client how he or she wants to take the medication. This offers some control and increases a sense of power over the situation. Clients must be monitored for desired and adverse effects of these agents, par-ticularly haloperidol, which can produce acute extrapyramidal side effects, such as acute dystonia.

4. Drugs previously discussed best manage pharmacological man-agement of acute agitation or aggressive behaviors. New stud-ies suggest that atypical neuroleptics, such as olanzapine and mood stabilizers, such as valproate are useful in treating chronic aggression.

Physical Interventions (Restraints and Seclusion)

Periodically, psychosocial and pharmacological interventions are inef-fective in controlling violent and aggressive behavior. When clients fail to respond to these interventions, clinicians must resort to physical interventions. Successful use of physical restraints or seclusion requires adequately trained staff who can initiate a plan and subdue the client safely. Before any decision about physical interventions is made, hospital security should be summoned to the area. Grove (1997) asserts that this must be *the first step* in the decision-making process. Normally, the arrival of security alerts the client that the staff is willing to initiate interventions that enable them to control the client's behavior.

Facilities must have policies and procedures for using physical interventions. Restraints are used as the last resort when clients are assessed as dangerous to themselves. Restraints may be used on a short-term basis so the clinician can administer medication, or longer if medications are contraindicated.

Table XVIII: Suggestions for Using Restraints

- At least 4 people should restrain the patient, while the 5th controls the client's head and prevents biting
- Explain to the client the purpose of being restrained
- Give the client a few seconds to comply, but do not negotiate
- As prearranged, the team applies the restraints, then moves the client to seclusion
- Staff should always be visible to reassure the client and alleviate feelings of helplessness
- Remove all dangerous objects from the client
- Raise the client's head while in restraints to minimize feelings of vulnerability and aspiration
- Initiate verbal interventions or rapid tranquilization
- Provide an opportunity for debriefing or allow the client to gain a perspective of the situation

Legal Considerations

1. Clinicians are facing more responsibilities and duties because of the rise in treating sicker and potentially violent clients. They have a professional, legal, and ethical responsibility to provide appropriate care and referrals for clients exhibiting aggressive and violent behavior.

147

2. *Mandatory reporting* of all known or suspected violent incidents help determine the magnitude of the problem.

3. Special rules, regulations and responsibilities exist for mental health clinicians who provide psychiatric emergency care. The standard of care provided by clinicians must be within the scope of their practice and consistent with individual state practice laws. Even so, when treatments go awry, the psychiatrist bears the burden of liability. Clinicians should provide care to clients exhibiting violent or aggressive behavior until they can be hospitalized, safely discharged or transferred to appropriate treatment centers.

4. Other legal and ethical issues that impact the care of violent clients involve the duty to warn and protect third parties at risk of harm from a client's action. Several states still hold that disclosures of any confidential nature violates the client's rights, while other state laws use more permissive language such as "may warn or protect," but do not require the clinicians to take action. However, Beck (1985) submits that the duty to protect third parties is currently a national standard of practice.

5. Legal considerations must direct the clinicians decision making process when determining the appropriate disposition and referrals. (*See* Chapter 5 for a more in-depth discussion of legal considerations.)

Disposition

1. Referrals and dispositions for the violent client should be based on the underlying causative factors and treatment planning. For instance, if the client's behavior arises from an underlying medical condition, such as delirium—hospitaliza-

tion is the referral of choice to further evaluate and treat the medical. The same holds true for the client who has a psychiatric disorder, such as bipolar disorder-manic episode, that requires medication stabilization and protection from potential harm to self and others.

2. Involuntary hospitalization is indicated when the client is a clear danger to self and others and refuses treatment. This referral also allows for further evaluation and treatment of the underlying condition that increases the client's level of dangerousness. The client with a history of chronic schizophrenia with acute exacerbation, who is a threat to himself or others, and refuses to be medicated is an example of a situation that warrants consideration for involuntary hospitalization.

3. If the client is medically and psychiatrically stable appropriate referrals may include residential crisis management, mobile crisis unit, psychotherapy day hospital or treatment and substance rehabilitation.

4. Other referrals for children and adolescents who are stable may include residential treatment, substance rehabilitation, family therapy, medication management.

Suggested Reading

Asnis, GM, Kaplan, ML, Hundorfean, G, Saeed, W (1997). Violence and homicidal behaviors in psychiatric disorders. *Psychiatric Clinics of North America, 20,* 405–425.

Beck, JC (1985). The psychotherapist and the violent patient: Recent case law. In JC Beck (ed.) *The Potentially Violent Patient and the Tarasoff Decision in Psychiatric Practice.* Washington, DC: American Psychiatric Press.

Citrome, L & Volavka, J (1999). Violent patients in the emergency setting. *Psychiatric Clinics of North America, 22,* 789–801.

Currier, GW & Allen, MH (2000). Physical and chemical restraint in psychiatric emergency service. *Psychiatric Services, 51,* 717–719.

Groves, JE (1997). Difficult patients. In NE Cassem; TA Stern; JF Rossenbaum; MS Jellinek (Eds.) *Massachusetts General Hospital Handbook of General Hospital Psychiatry, 4th edition* (pp. 337–366). St. Louis: Mosby.

Lagomasino, I; Daly, R & Stoudemire, A (1999). Medical assessment of patients presenting with psychiatric symptoms in the emergency setting. *Psychiatric Clinics of North America, 22,* 819–850.

Otto, RK (2000). Assessing and managing violence risk in outpatient settings. *Journal of Clinical Psychology, 56,* 1239–1262.

Steadman, HJ; Mulvey, E; Monahan, J; Robbins, P; Appelbaum, PS; Grisso, T; Roth, LH & Silver, E (1998). Violence by people discharged from acute psychiatric inpatient facilities and by others in the same neighborhoods. *Archives of General Psychiatry, 55,* 393–401.

Tardiff, K (1998). Usual diagnoses among violent patients. *Psychiatric Clinics of North America, 21,* 567–576.

Borderline Personality Disorder and Self-Injurious Behaviors

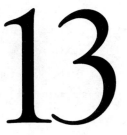

1. Clients diagnosed with borderline personality disorder (BPD) are among the most disliked and high users of psychiatric emergency services. They often present with an array of symptoms, such as major depressive episode, posttraumatic stress disorder, panic disorder, and suicidal or self-injurious behaviors in the context of an interpersonal crisis.

2. Women with BPD comprise a large proportion of clients who make repeated visits to emergency psychiatric settings. Major reasons for seeking these services include suicidal and parasuicidal behaviors, intense emotional and behavioral disturbances and intense rage.

3. Suicide attempts and other self-injurious behaviors, such as drug overdose and bodily cutting, are common in these

clients and they are the basis of their visits to emergency psychiatric settings. Suicide attempts are usually associated with forestalling the possibility of a physical abandonment or relationship break-up.

4. *Self-injurious* behaviors include suicidal behaviors and self-mutilation. Self-mutilation refers to a deliberate alteration or destruction of body tissue without the conscious intent of suicide. Characteristics of self-mutilation also include low lethality and a sporadic or repetitive course. Examples of these behaviors range from major, such as castration, to stereotypical (i.e., head banging). The most common type found in clients with BPD is superficial or moderate type.

Evaluation

1. Clients with BPD also present themselves as emotionally and behaviorally overwhelmed and disorganized. Clinicians should provide an empathetic and structured setting that enables them to form a therapeutic relationship, develop and maintain clear and appropriate boundaries, discern treatment goals and foster the client's sense of self-competence and functioning.

2. Clients with BPD are frequently unreliable historians and it is imperative that clinicians gather as much corroborative data as possible from vast sources.

3. When assessing clients with BPD it is imperative for clinicians to pay attention to their own feelings during the interviewing process. Common reactions to these clients include anger, frustration, rescue fantasies, hopelessness, and helplessness, which can be clues about the client's inner states. Recognizing

these states can be useful in guiding questions and comments during the assessment process.

4. All suicidal threats or gestures in these clients must be taken serious and thoroughly assessed. An important disposition issue involves assessing the client's ability to manage his or her safety without external interventions. Clinicians must deal with their own reactions to perceived manipulation and assess these clients for their risk of dangerousness to themselves and others.

5. *Differential diagnosis* involves ruling out underlying medical, psychiatric, such as mood and anxiety disorders, and substance-related disorders.

Physical Examination

Physical findings in these clients are associated with underlying causative factors that prompted their visit to the emergency setting. Signs of self-mutilation or self-injurious behaviors may also be found on physical examination.

Mental Status Examination

- Intense anxiety
- Suicidal threats, gestures, self-injurious behaviors
- Impulsivity
- Agitation
- Depression
- Argumentive
- Hyperarousal

Management

Management goals for the client with BPD are symptomatic and relate to the client's present emotional and physical state. Common behaviors in these clients also include manipulation and staff splitting. Management strategies should be brief and structured.

Psychosocial Intervention

1. Rouse (1994) suggests that the psychiatric emergency setting should be a "holding environment" that offers: 1) empathy; 2) limit setting; 3) consistency of treatment and boundaries; and 4) communication between the client and various health care providers.

2. Assess the client and family member's health teaching needs and provide information.

3. Clinicians can use the following strategies for dealing with manipulative behaviors:

   • Confront the client and describe the unacceptable behavior

   • Convey feelings and thoughts assertively

   • Suggest alternative ways to get needs met

   • Ignore manipulative behavior when possible

   • Redirect attention on the client's behavior when an attempt to focus on other's behavior occurs

   • Provide clear and direct communication

   • Set consistent limits and provide role modeling

   • Encourage expression of feelings and avoid engaging in arguments and defensiveness

   • Point out manipulative behavior and consequences

Pharmacological Interventions

Target symptoms for pharmacological interventions should follow the principles of a psychiatric emergency and based on the client's presenting symptoms.

Disposition

1. Because of the complexity of BPD, clients with this disorder require diverse interventions, including hospitalization when the client is medically or psychiatrically unstable.

2. Refer client back to primary therapist and contact this individual whenever possible. Sometimes the client "acts out" when the therapist is on vacation.

3. Give the client a community appointment for follow-up. Review with the client and significant others instructions for dealing with future emergencies, being alone, and crisis situations.

4. Community referrals are contingent on the client's presentation and may include dialectical behavioral therapy (DBT), medication management to treat Axis I diagnosis, such as posttraumatic stress disorder, mood disorders, and impulsivity behaviors. Treatment using DBT typically consists of a 3-month inpatient program prior to long-term treatment. According to Linehan this model is designed for outpatient treatment of chronically suicidal clients with BPD. Crisis hot lines, crisis residential centers and substance rehabilitation facilities are also helpful resources.

5. Referrals for adolescents and their families should include family therapies, health education and support groups.

Suggested Reading

Antai-Otong, D (2003). Treatment considerations for the patient with borderline personality disorder. *Nursing Clinics of North America, 38,* 101–109.

Bohus, H; Haaf, B; Simms, T; Limberger, MF; Schmahl, C; Unckel, C; Lieb, K & Linehan, MM (2004). Effectiveness of inpatient dialectical behavior therapy for borderline personality disorder: A controlled study. *Behavioral Research Therapy, 42,* 487–499.

Gunderson, JG (2001). *Borderline personality disorder: A clinical guide.* Washington, DC: American Psychiatric Publishing.

Linehan, MM; Heard, HL & Armstrong, HE (1993). Naturalistic follow-up of a behavioral treatment for chronically parasuicidal borderline patients. *Archives of General Psychiatry, 50,* 971–974.

Linehan, MM; Schmidt, III, H; Dimeff, LA; et al (1999). Dialectical behavior therapy for patients with borderline personality disorder and drug dependence. *American Journal of Addiction, 8,* 279–292.

Koerner, K & Linehan, MM (2000). Research on dialectical behavior therapy for patients with borderline personality disorder. *Psychiatric Clinics of North America, 23,* 151–167.

Rouse, JD (1994). Borderline and other dramatic personality disorders in the psychiatric service. *Psychiatric Annals, 24,* 598–602.

Sexual Assault 14

Epidemiology and Prevalence

1. An epidemiological study shows a prevalence of 9.2% of women and 1% of men reported a history of sexual assault.

2. Sexual assault or rape is a crime of controlling victims with violent, nonconsensual sex acts.

3. Studies also reveal that women who reports a history of physical or sexual assault have significantly higher rates of general medical health complaints ranging from gynecological and gastrointestinal symptoms, chronic pain syndrome, sexual dysfunction and functional disturbances. These data also confirm that sexual assault survivors are more likely to visit a health care provider with physical complaints than a mental health professional.

4. Results across several epidemiological studies indicate that sexual and physical assault are more associated with a high risk of post-traumatic stress disorder (PTSD) than other traumatic events. Lifetime rates of PTSD among women who survive sexual assault ranges from an estimated 30% to more than 50%. Risk factors for PTSD comprise previous history of assaults, perception of the survivor that she could be seriously injured or killed during the assault.

5. Other psychiatric disorders associated with sexual assault include depression, panic disorder or panic attacks and increased rates of suicidal ideations and attempts.

Evaluation

1. Upon arrival to the ED, clinicians must triage the sexual assault survivor as a priority and treat life-threatening injuries according to legal protocols.

2. Medical clearance must be quickly determined.

3. *Safety and social support* are major priorities for helping the sexual assault survivor. Provide a quiet and private room for interviewing and allow significant others to accompany the client during the assessment.

4. Major priorities of the sexual assault protocol include minimizing the psychological and physical impact of trauma while expanding the collection of forensic evidence (Young, Bracken, Goddard, et. al, 1992).

5. Common stress reactions associated with sexual assault include disorganization, shock and disbelief, and denial. Rape trauma syndrome usually occurs within 24 to 72 hours and includes the following:

- emotional numbness
- disbelief
- severe anxiety
- anger
- humiliation and self-blame
- depression

Other sexual assault survivors may exhibit a sense of outward calmness, compliance and talkativeness. Clients exhibiting these symptoms are just as overwhelmed and distressed as those who exhibit the former symptoms.

Symptoms of the *chronic rape syndrome* generally occur within months to years after the incident and include:

- major depressive episode
- panic disorder
- PTSD
- suicide attempts or gestures
- sexual disturbances
- substance abuse or dependence

6. The focus of the assessment process of sexual assault victims must begin with a brief *focused approach.* Assessment questions should be *concise, simply worded and brief.* Afford a private room and avoid intrusiveness. Provide explanations for queries and stress that they are routine and designed to provide quality care. Anticipate the client's difficulty in concentrating and answering questions

7. During the early phase of the acute rape syndrome, the client often appears in a daze and has problems concentrating and modulating their emotional and behavioral responses. Because of these reactions, clinicians may need to repeat questions more than once.

   a. Avoid retraumatizing the client by rushing or hurrying the client to answer questions

   b. Allow the client to answer questions at her or his own pace.

   c. Encourage the client to express feelings and thoughts about the incident

   d. Reassure the client and family members about the normalcy of their reactions

8. Efforts to *normalize* the client's responses must be an integral part of the assessment process and treatment. Assess the client and family members' knowledge about sexual assault and trauma and health teaching needs. Health teaching about normal or expected reactions and validation of the clients cognitive, behavioral, and emotional reactions provides an accepting, safe and supportive environment.

9. Clinicians working with the sexual assault survivor must also be cognizant of their own reactions, particularly if they are also sexual assault survivors and have not resolved their own grief issues. Unresolved grief issues in the clinician will impact the assessment process and interfere with an objective approach and intervention.

10. Assessing the client's global responses also include assessing and treating existing injuries. A female provider is preferred to allay the client's anxiety and fears during the actual physical examination. All physical injuries should be documented. Rape protocols should be followed. Assess for other psychiatric and substance-related disorders. Inquire about last menstrual period, contraceptives, and last date of consensual sexual contact. Other gynecological questions include the time of the assault, and whether the client has showered, douched, changed clothes, urinated or defecated since the assault.

Physical Examination

Serious physical injuries should be referred for medical evaluation and treatment. Most sexual survivors sustain perineal and vaginal tearing. The examination should include documentation of physical findings and include type of injuries and trauma, including lacerations, stab wounds, bites, contusions, pregnancy and sexually transmitted diseases

(STDs). The physician in the ED is likely to order a battery of diagnostic studies including pregnancy test, screening for STDs, hepatitis, B and refer for human immunodeficiency virus (HIV). Findings from the pelvic examination should also be documented.

Mental Status Examination

Emotional

- anxiety
- confusion
- emotional numbness
- anger
- depression
- distrust

Behavioral

- aggression
- avoidance
- alienation
- social isolation or aloofness
- substance misuse
- suicidal gestures/attempts

Cognitive

- distrust of men
- loss of safety
- loss of independence
- loss of faith
- "dazed state"

Management

Major treatment centers on ensuring safety, restoring self-esteem, alleviating guilt and shame, establishing trust, and managing anger effectively.

Psychosocial Interventions

1. Approach the client using an accepting and nonjudgmental approach
2. Ensure safety
3. Provide crisis intervention
4. Inform client that recovery begins immediately
5. Provide reassurance that reactions are normal
6. Encourage client to take control of life and improve safety by obtaining medical examination, staying with a friend, reporting the assault, and changing the door locks
7. Be cognizant of laws governing sexual assault and document all clinical findings
8. *Family interventions* should include:

   - assessing their response to the client
   - determining if they are a source of support
   - discussing ways they can be supportive
   - stressing the importance of listening to and believing the client
   - educating them about normal reactions
   - discouraging the from isolating or rescuing the client
   - encouraging them to express their feelings and thoughts about the incident

Pharmacological Interventions

1. Pharmacological interventions are limited to intense anxiety reactions, such as panic attacks. Benzodiazepines, such as clonazepam (Klonopin) may be useful in managing acute anxiety reactions and aggressive behavior.

Legal Considerations

1. Follow legal protocols for sexual assault
2. Document pertinent clinical findings including physical and mental status exams
3. Document specific information about the alleged assault to be reported to law enforcement
4. Document pertinent information from the assessment including the date, time and location of the assault
5. Record all physical injuries or pain described by the client

Disposition

1. Provide information about community referrals, rape crisis counseling or other crisis centers or agencies
2. Make appropriate treatment referrals for comorbid psychiatric, such as depression and PTSD or substance-related disorders
3. Hospitalization is indicated for the client who is medically or psychiatrically unstable (i.e., life-threatening injuries, suicidal)

Suggested Reading

Boudreaux, E; Kilpatrick, DG; Resnick, HS; Best, CL & Saunders, BE (1998). Criminal victimization, posttraumatic stress disorder, and comorbid psychopathology among a community sample of women. *Journal of Traumatic Stress, 11,* 665–678.

Falsetti, SA & Resnick, HS (1997). Trauma, posttraumatic stress disorder, and panic attacks: Frequency, severity, and implications for treatment. *Journal of Traumatic Stress, 10,* 683–689.

Golding, JM (1996). Sexual assault history and limitations in physical functioning in two general population samples. *Research in Nursing and Health, 19,* 33–44.

Goodman, LA; Koss, MP & Russo, NF (1993). Violence against women: Physical and mental health effects: Part I: Research findings. *Applied and Preventive Psychology, 2,* 79–89.

Kaysen, D; Resick, PA & Wise (2003). Living in danger: The impact of chronic traumatization and the traumatic context on post traumatic stress disorder. *Trauma and Violence Abuse, 4,* 247–264.

Kessler, RC; Sonnega, A; Bromet, E; Hughes, M & Nelson, CB (1995). Posttraumatic stress disorder in the National Comorbidity Survey. *Archives of General Psychiatry, 52,* 1048–1060.

Najavits, LM, Sonn, J, Walsh, M & Weiss, RD (2004). Domestic violence in women with PTSD and substance abuse. *Addictive Behavior, 29,* 707–715.

Resnick, HS; Acierno, R & Kilpatrick, DG (1997). Health impact of interpersonal violence 2: Medical and mental health outcomes. *Behavioral Medicine, 23,* 65–78.

Smith-McKenna, L & Grant, C (2003). The client who survives violence. In D Antai-Otong (ed.) *Psychiatric Nursing: Biological and Behavioral Concepts* (pp. 661–690). Clifton Park, NY: Delmar Thomson Learning.

Street, AE & Arias, I (2001). Psychological abuse and posttraumatic stress disorder in battered women: examining the roles of shame and guilt. *Violence and Victimization, 16,* 65–78.

Young, WW; Bracken, AC; Goddard, MA & the New Hampshire Committee: Sexual Assault Medical Examination Protocol Project Committee (1992). Sexual assault: Review of a national protocol for forensic and medical evaluation. *Obstetrical and Gynecological, 80,* 878–883.

Domestic Violence 15

Epidemiology and Prevalence

1. Domestic violence is a pervasive and devastating societal problem. More than 1.5 million women are beaten by their partners annually in the United States (Straus & Gelles, 1990; Straus & Gelles, 1986).

2. Battering and physical violence encompasses more than just physical violence. The chief intent of batterers is intimidation and control of another. Many batterers use threats, taunts, progressive social isolation, sexual assault, and humiliation. Psychological abuse occurs more frequently and often precedes physical abuse.

3. Other researchers submit that at least their partners will physically assault a third of all women during the lifetime. Even more alarming, is that women are more likely to be killed by their male partners than any category of perpetrators (Browne, 1993; Browne & Williams, 1993).

4. The disturbing high prevalence of domestic violence and the marked psychological and physical aftermath of both victims

and perpetrators are sufficient to warrant clinical assessment for spousal abuse.

5. Domestic violence is a broad definition that comprises an array of behaviors and behavior patterns, ranging from a single incident of slapping or grabbing during a heated argument to a continuous and pervasive pattern of severe battering and coercion. Although the literature shows that men are usually the perpetrators, the possibility of women batterers also exists.

6. Risk factors for domestic violence include:

   • violence in the family of origin
   • previous aggressive behavior
   • interpersonal conflict
   • alcohol use
   • pregnancy
   • relationship termination

Evaluation

1. Most women who are battered seek treatment in the ED for medical problems rather than trauma, suggesting the need to intervene as soon as feasible and routine screening for domestic violence.

2. When interviewing or assessing survivors of domestic violence, clinicians should avoid an overly directive or controlling approach or a lack of empathy. This approach reinforces victimization and often results in denial of abuse. Clinicians are more likely to establish rapport and validate the client's expe-

rience by using a supportive and nonjudgmental approach that takes concerns seriously and affords care, information, and guidance. Avoid probing questions about abuse and be cognizant of emotional and physical cues, such as low self-esteem, poor eye contact and hesitant and monotone speech.

3. A supportive and safe approach involves creating a confidential environment conducive to disclosure. Many of these women feel ashamed and embarrassed and find it difficult to share their experiences. However, they are often relieved to finally be able to talk about the abuse. Clinicians can minimize tension and anxiety by expressing an interest and encouraging a dialogue of the prospect of abuse. Perform the assessment confidentially, in the *absence of the perpetrator (abuser)*.

4. Assess the client's safety level. Prior to asking questions about safety, inform the client that these are routine questions.

   a. Questions should center on the mnemonic SAFE: S—stress and safety, A—afraid/abused, F—friends/family, E—emergency plan (Asher, 1993)

   b. Questions, such as "are you or your children safe at home?" If the client admits to domestic violence, other questions are also useful in determining safety, such as "Do you have a safety plan?" "What will you do the next time your spouse becomes violent?"

5. Assessing clients for abuse as both a survivor and perpetrator should be a routine part of the psychobiological assessment. *Awareness* is the heart to diagnosis, it should *guide* interventions with a subsequent *empowerment* and ultimate survivor *safety* (Ortega, 1998).

6. *Differential diagnosis* involves thoroughly reviewing the clients medical history and current symptoms and injuries. Inspect the client's injuries, observe interaction between the client and spouse (when present) and interview each partner separately. Routine laboratory and diagnostic studies, including pregnancy tests and toxicology screens, provide invaluable information about the client's current physical and mental status. Assess the client's level of dangerousness to self and others. The following questions may elicit pertinent information that helps rule out medical and psychiatric or substance-related disorders:

- What happened to cause these injuries?
- Do you feel afraid of your spouse/partner?
- Are you safe at home?
- Has your spouse hurt you in the past?
- Where does abuse usually occur? Home? Outside the home?
- What options do you have?

Physical Examination

Life-threatening injuries must be quickly assessed and medically managed. The physical examination must be comprehensive. All physical injuries must be documented accurately with a body map or photographs for current and potential legal reasons. Physical assault occurs intermittently and physical findings characteristic of domestic violence include:

- multiple sites of injuries at various healing stages including fractures and bruises

- imprints left by the tool of destruction
- lacerations, contusions of the breasts, chest, genitalia (areas usually hidden and more difficult to detect)
- fractures
- soft tissue injuries to the head and neck
- burns
- headache
- back pain
- chronic irritable bowel syndrome
- facial trauma
- sensory loss (hearing, vision, and concentration problems)
- bladder infections
- anal tearing
- sexually transmitted diseases (STDs)
- abdominal bleeding
- bruises around the wrists, ankles or neck (secondary to being physically restrained)

Mental Status Examination

The acute and chronic impact of spousal abuse is phenomenal and produces an array of emotions. Posttraumatic and other anxiety and mood disorders are common consequences of domestic violence. Battered women often experience shame, low-self esteem and the following are characteristic findings on the mental status exam:

- poor eye contact
- shock

- disbelief
- confusion
- terror
- fear
- anger
- depression
- anxiety
- suicidal ideations, attempts, suicide
- homicide
- panic attacks
- apologizes excessively
- unkempt appearance
- a sense of helplessness
- hyperarousal and/or easily startled

Psychosocial Interventions

(Previously discussed in the Evaluation section of this chapter)

1. Inform client that she is not the cause of the abuse nor does she deserve to be abused.

2. Provide information about community social support services.

3. Encourage her to develop a safety plan for herself and children.

4. Encourage her to keep important papers, documents, phone numbers, and cash in a safe place accessible outside the home.

5. Recognize that the woman knows when it is safe to leave her abusive partner.

Pharmacological Interventions

1. Based on client's presentation including the presence of acute psychiatric symptoms, such as acute panic attacks.

Legal Considerations

1. Be cognizant of federal and state laws associated with domestic violence. Many states are adopting mandatory reporting laws.
2. Communicate the diagnosis of abuse to others only with written consent from the abused survivor. Sharing this information with the perpetrator and others may jeopardize the survivor's life and safety.

Disposition

1. Refer to medical triage for evaluation of life-threatening injuries
2. Hospitalize if client is an imminent danger to self or others or is psychiatrically unstable
3. Make appropriate community referrals for battered women, including 24-hour hotlines, legal advocates and battered woman's advocate
4. Refer to community mental health centers for crisis intervention, medication management and psychotherapy when appropriate
5. Provide information about The National Coalition Against Domestic Violence provides information about local community and state services and other resources (1-800-799-SAFE)

6. Arrange for admission or transfer to battered woman's shelter or safe place when life-threatening situation exists

Suggested Reading

Ashur, M (1993). Asking questions about domestic violence: SAFE questions. JAMA, *269*, 2367

Browne, A (1993). Violence against women by male partners: Prevalences, outcomes, and policy implications. *American Psychologist, 48*, 1077–1087.

Browne, A & Williams KR (1993). Gender, intimacy, and lethal violence: Trends from 1976–1987. *Gender and Society, 7*, 78–98.

Campbell, JC & Lewandowski, LA (1997). Mental and physical health effects of intimae partner violence on women and children. *Psychiatric Clinics of North America, 20*, 353–374.

Curry, MA & Harvey, SM (1998). Stress related to domestic violence during pregnancy and infant birth weight. In JC Campbell, et al (Eds.) *Empowering Survivors of Abuse: Health Care For Battered Women and Their Children*. Sage series on *Volence Against Women* (pp.98–108). Thousand Oaks, CA: Sage Publications.

Holmes, WC & Slap, GB (1998). Sexual abuse of boys: Definition, prevalence, correlates, sequelae and management. JAMA, *280*, 1855–1862.

McFarlane, J, Parker, B, & Soeken, K (1995). Abuse during pregnancy: Frequency, severity, perpetrator, and risk factors of homicide. *Public Health Nursing, 12*, 284–289.

Muelleman, RA, Lenaghan, PA, & Pakieser, RA (1996). Battered women: Injury locations and types. *Annals of Emergency Medicine, 28*, 486–492.

Ortega, C (1998). Family violence and elder abuse. In JM Howell, M Alteiri, AS Jagoda, JE Prescott, JL Scott, & TO Stair (Eds.)

Emergency Medicine, Volume II (pp. 1626–1632). Philadelphia: WB Saunders.

Sachs, CJ, Baraff, LJ, & Peek, C (1998). Need for law enforcement in cases of intimate partner violence in a university ED. *American Journal of Emergency Medicine, 16,* 60–63.

Smith-McKenna, L & Grant, C (2003). The client who survives violence. In D Antai-Otong (ed.) *Psychiatric Nursing: Biological and Behavioral Concepts* (pp. 661–690). Clifton Park, NY: Delmar Thomson Learning.

Straus, MA & Gelles, RJ (1990). *Physical violence in American families: Risk factors and adaptation to violence in 8,145 families.* New Brunswick, NJ: Transaction.

Straus, MA & Gelles, RJ (1986) societal change and change in family violence from 1975 to 1985 as revealed by two national surveys. *Journal of Marriage and the Family, 48,* 465–479.

Index

STUDY PACKAGE
CONTINUING EDUCATION
CREDIT INFORMATION

PSYCHIATRIC EMERGENCIES

Thank you for choosing PESI Healthcare as your continuing education provider. Our goal is to provide you with current, accurate and practical information from the most experienced and knowledgeable speakers and authors.

Listed below are the continuing education credit(s) currently available for this self-study package. ***Please note, your state licensing board dictates whether self study is an acceptable form of continuing education. Please refer to your state rules and regulations.*

Counselors: PESI HealthCare, LLC is recognized by the National Board for Certified Counselors to offer continuing education for National Certified Counselors. Provider #: 5896. We adhere to NBCC Continuing Education Guidelines. These self-study materials qualify for 3.5 contact hours.

Psychologists: PESI is approved by the American Psychological Association to offer continuing education for psychologists. PESI maintains responsibility for the material. PESI is offering this self-study activity for 3.5 hours of continuing education credit. PESI Healthcare, LLC maintains responsibility for the program.

Social Workers: PESI HealthCare, 1030, is approved as a provider for social work continuing education by the Association of Social Work Boards (ASWB), (540-829-6880) through the Approved Continuing Education (ACE) program. Licensed Social Workers should contact their individual state boards to determine self-study approval and to review continuing education requirements for licensure renewal. Social Workers will receive 3.5 continuing education clock hours for completing this self-study material.

Addiction Counselors: PESI HealthCare, LLC is a Provider approved by NAADAC Approved Education Provider Program. Provider #: 366. These self-study materials qualify for 4.0 contact hours.

Nurses: PESI HealthCare, LLC, Eau Claire is an approved provider of continuing nursing education by the Wisconsin Nurses Association Continuing Education Approval Program Committee, an accredited approver by the American Nurses Credentialing Center's Commission on Accreditation. This approval is accepted and/or recognized by all state nurses associations that adhere to the ANA criteria for accreditation. This learner directed educational activity qualifies for 4.2 contact hours. PESI Healthcare certification: CA #06538.

Procedures: 1. Read book.
                    2. Complete the post-test/evaluation form and mail it along with payment (if necessary) to the address on the form.

Your completed test/evaluation will be graded. If you receive a passing score (80% and above), you will be mailed a certificate of successful completion with earned continuing education credits. If you do not pass the post-test, you will be sent a letter indicating areas of deficiency, references to the appropriate sections of the manual for review and your post-test. The post-test must be resubmitted and receive a passing grade before credit can be awarded.

If you have any questions, please feel free to contact our customer service department at 1-800-843-7763.

PESI HealthCare, LLC
200 SPRING ST. STE B, P.O. BOX 1000
EAU CLAIRE, WI 54702-1000

Product Number: SAM006410   **CE Release Date:** 7/13/04

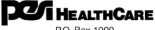 **HEALTHCARE**

P.O. Box 1000
Eau Claire, WI 54702
(800) 843-7763

Psychiatric Emergencies

ZNT006410

This home study package includes CONTINUING EDUCATION FOR ONE PERSON: complete & return this original post/test evaluation form.

ADDITIONAL PERSONS interested in receiving credit may photocopy this form, complete and return with a payment of $25.00 per person CE fee. A certificate of successful completion will be mailed to you.

For office use only
Rcvd. _____
Graded _____
Cert. mld. _____

C.E. Fee: **$25**

Credit card # _____

Exp. Date _____

Signature _____

V-Code* _____ (*MC/VISA/Discover: last 3-digit # on signature panel on back of card.) (*American Express: 4-digit # above account # on face of card.)

Mail to: PESI HealthCare, PO Box 1000, Eau Claire, WI 54702, or
Fax to: PESI HealthCare (800) 675-5026 (fax all pages)

Name (please print): _____ _____ _____
LAST   FIRST   M.I.

Address: _____

City: _____ State: _____ Zip: _____

Daytime Phone: _____

Signature: _____

• Date you completed the PESI HC Tape/Manual Independent Package: _____

• Actual time (# of hours) taken to complete this offering: _____ hours

LEARNING OBJECTIVES

How well did we do in presenting the following objectives?

	Excellent				**Poor**
Designing a plan of care for patients presenting with a psychiatric emergency.	5	4	3	2	1
Compiling populations at risk for suicide and homicide.	5	4	3	2	1
Discussing major verbal de-escalation and escape techniques in potentially violent patients.	5	4	3	2	1
Describing measures that may reduce the aftermath of critical incidents in health care professionals.	5	4	3	2	1
Distinguishing medical and psychiatric causes of psychosis.	5	4	3	2	1
Describing psychiatric emergencies associated with psychotic disorders.	5	4	3	2	1
Differentiating symptoms of delirium and dementia.	5	4	3	2	1
Assessing intoxication and withdrawal symptoms associated with alcohol and other psychoactive drugs.	5	4	3	2	1
Analyzing symptoms and treatment of acute anxiety and mood disorders.	5	4	3	2	1

POST-TEST QUESTIONS

1. When working with clients in psychiatric emergency situations, it is imperative for the nurse to maintain a safe exit.

   True or **False**

2. Most patients who kill themselves have a psychiatric disorder.

   True or **False**

3. Some medical emergencies are associated are misdiagnosed as psychiatric conditions, especially if there is a history of mental illness.

   True or **False**

4. Which of the following is likely to increase the risk of suicide among youth?

   a. History of a mood disorder
   b. Positive family history of suicide
   c. Situational stress
   d. All of the above

5. Which of the following cluster indicate mania or bipolar disorder, manic, most recent episode?

   a. Psychomotor retardation, concentration difficulties, visual disturbances
   b. Talkativeness, racing thoughts, intrusiveness, rapid speech, increased energy
   c. Auditory hallucinations, aloofness, suspiciousness, marked anhedonia
   d. Visual hallucinations, time distortions, paranoia, suspiciousness

6. What is the most accurate statement about pharmacological interventions for acute psychosis?

   a. Typical antipsychotic medications are less effective than atypical agents.
   b. Oral administration is the best route when a client exhibits acute symptoms and agitation.
   c. Atypical antipsychotic agents are less likely to produce movement disorders than typical agents.
   d. The treatment of substance-induced psychosis is the same regardless of the drug.

7. Untreated or inadequately treated panic disorder is associated with a high suicide risk.

   True or **False**

8. Hypervigilance, sleep disturbances, intrusive thoughts, startle response and avoidance behaviors are hallmark symptoms of social anxiety disorder or social phobia.

   True or **False**

9. Which of the following is most likely to be prescribed for unipolar major depression?

   a. Tricyclic antidepressants

   b. Novel antidepressants, such SSRIs, venlafaxine, bupropion

   c. Benzodiazepines

   d. Mood stabilizers, such as lithium and depakote

For additional forms and information on other PESI products, contact:
**Customer Service; PESI HEALTHCARE; P.O. Box 1000; Eau Claire, WI 54702
(Toll Free, 7 a.m.–5 p.m. central time, 800-843-7763).**
www.pesihealthcare.com

**Thank you for your comments.
We strive for excellence and we value your opinion.**

Professional Resources Available from PESI HealthCare

Resources for Mental Health Professionals

Addiction, Progression & Recovery, by Dale Kesten, LCSW, LADC

Assessing and Treating Trauma and PTSD, by Linda Schupp, Ph.D

Borderline Personality Disorder—Struggling, Understanding, Succeeding, by Colleen E. Warner, Psy.D

Case Management Handbook for Clinicians, by Rand L. Kannenberg, MA

Clinicians Update on the Treatment and Management of Anxiety Disorders, by Deborah Antai-Otong, MS, RN, CNS, NP, CS, FAAN

Collaborative Healing: A Shorter Therapy Approach for Survivors of Sexual Abuse, by Mark Hirschfeld, LCSW-C, BCD & Jill B. Cody, MA

Delirium—The Mistaken Confusion, by Debra Cason-McNeeley, MSN, RNCS

Depression and Other Mood Disorders, by Deborah Antai-Otong, MS, RN, CNS, NP, CS, FAAN

Effective Strategies for Helping Couples and Families, by John S. Carpenter

Grief: Normal, Complicated, Traumatic, by Linda Schupp, Ph.D

Psychiatric Emergencies, by Deborah Antai-Otong, MS, RN, CNS, NP, CS, FAAN

Sociotherapy for Sociopaths: Resocial Group, by Rand L. Kannenberg, MA

Resources for Nurses & Other Healthcare Professionals

Heart and Lung Sounds Reference Library (Audio CD), by Diane Wrigley, PA-C

Infection Control and Emerging Infectious Diseases, by William Barry Inman

Legal and Ethical Standards for Nurses, by Sheryl Feutz-Harter

Managing Urinary Incontinence (Audio CD), by Carol Ann White, RN, MS, ANPC, GNPC

Mechanisms and Treatment of Disease: Pathophysiology—A Plain English Approach, by Mikel A. Rothenberg, MD

Oral Medication and Insulin Therapies: A Practical Guide for Reaching Diabetes Target Goals, by Charlene Freeman

Subclinical Signs of Impending Doom (Audio CD), by Carol Whiteside, RN, PhD(c)

Understanding X-Rays—A Plain English Approach, by Mikel A. Rothenberg

**To order these or other PESI HealthCare products
or to receive information about our national seminars,
please call 800-843-7763**

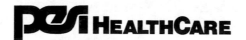

www.pesihealthcare.com